30-MINUTE WEIGHT LOSS
COOKBOOK

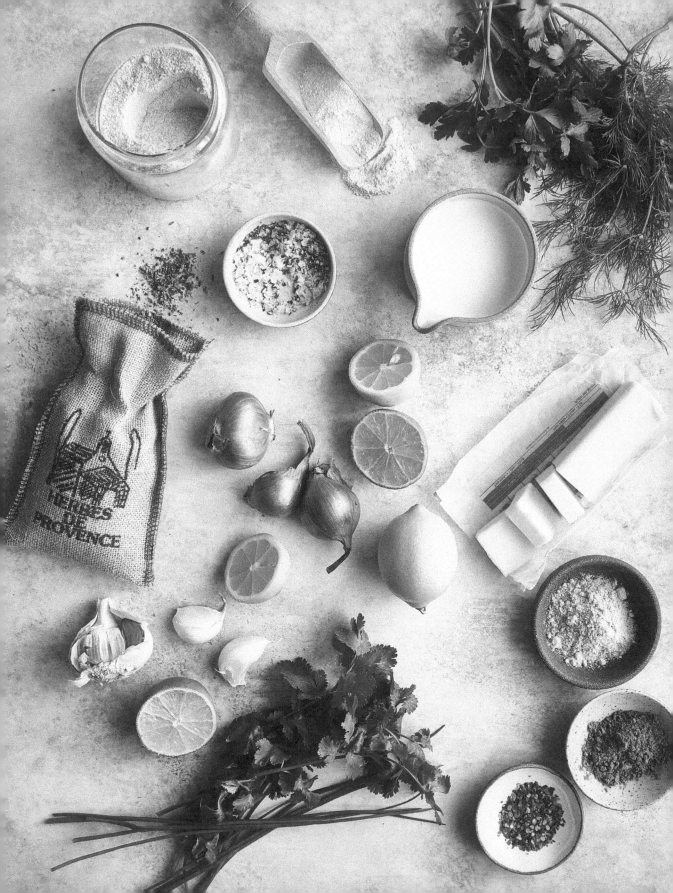

30-MINUTE WEIGHT LOSS COOKBOOK

100+ Quick and Easy Recipes for Sustainable Weight Loss

MANDY ENRIGHT, MS, RDN, RYT

ROCKRIDGE
PRESS

For general information on our other products and services or to obtain technical support, please contact our Customer Care Department within the United States at (866) 744-2665, or outside the United States at (510) 253-0500.

Rockridge Press publishes its books in a variety of electronic and print formats. Some content that appears in print may not be available in electronic books, and vice versa.

Interior and Cover Designer: Heather Krakora
Art Producer: Meg Baggott
Editor: Claire Yee
Production Editor: Ruth Sakata Corley
Production Manager: Riley Hoffman

Cover photo ©2021 Annie Martin; Hélène Dujardin, pp. ii, x, 156; Ewgenija Schall/StockFood USA, p 21; Zuzanna Ploch/StockFood USA, p 38; News Life Media/StockFood USA, p 56; Nadine Greeff/Stocksy United, p 72; Nicky Walsh/Gräfe & Unzer Verlag/Stockfood, p 82; Darren Muir, p 90; Cameron Whitman/Stocksy United, p 108; Meike Bergmann/StockFood USA, p 126; Mondadori Portfolio/StockFood USA, p 132; Great Stock!/StockFood USA, p 142. Author photo courtesy of Claire Sheprow/FindOrion Photography

ISBN: Print 978-1-64876-655-8
eBook 978-1-64876-154-6
R0

To Joe –
Here's to another chapter in the
#AdventuresOfTacoAndMandy.
Thanks for being my PIC
on this crazy journey called life.

CONTENTS

INTRODUCTION

Landing my dream job as an advertising executive in New York City after college turned out to be a nightmare for my health and weight. I was working overtime, eating meals at my desk after starving myself most of the day, ordering takeout for dinner, and never making any time for myself. I wasn't making *myself* a priority. It wasn't until I started putting my health first that I was able to make real and sustainable changes—to the point that I decided to leave advertising and become a registered dietitian.

I wasn't any less busy when I went back to school. In addition to being a full-time student, I was teaching fitness classes part-time, planning a wedding, trying to find time to get in shape for said wedding, and taking on the primary cooking responsibilities for me and my fiancé. Thirty-minute meals became essential, because most days that was all the time I had to cook—a far cry from the home I grew up in, where my mom made just about every meal from scratch.

During this time, I had one goal for my wedding: look fabulous on the big day, but not starve myself to make it happen. I was able to lose weight for my wedding without ever once going on a crazy "wedding diet." To do this, I went back to the basics of weight management: food and movement.

I concentrated on the quality and quantity of foods I was eating, instead of counting calories and holding myself to daily weigh-ins. I incorporated more vegetables and lean proteins, while also enjoying sweet treats and wine in moderation. I didn't skip any meals, so I didn't get hangry or overeat. I felt great and I wasn't stressed out about how I got there. And unlike most diets, where the wedding (or other event) is the end goal, it never occurred to me to stop my eating style after the wedding, because it had become habit. I felt good and didn't want to stop feeling that way. I had established a sustainable eating lifestyle based around quick, simple, delicious meals, and my new husband was on the train with me.

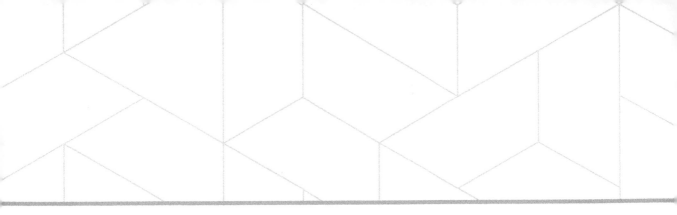

Life hasn't become any less hectic since then. Those 30-minute meals are still essential for our lifestyle, health, and keeping our weight in check. I don't want to spend all my free time in the kitchen cooking meals, and dining out all the time is not ideal for our household budget or weight. Cooking at home on a regular basis allows us to truly enjoy ourselves the one or two times a week we eat out.

I'm still not a calorie counter, and I don't encourage my clients to count calories, either. Counting calories isn't important if you're making the effort to eat the right foods and take control of your meals. That's where this book comes into play.

The practice of eating healthy to manage your weight shouldn't cause added stress in your life. You don't have to spend your entire night after a long day at work cooking. Heck, you shouldn't have to spend a precious weekend day in the kitchen for hours, either. I also don't recommend eating out all the time with meals you can't control ingredient-wise or portion-wise. The only weight loss happening there is in your wallet.

Busy friends, I created this book with you in mind, because that's my lifestyle, too. This book is loaded with fast, healthy, tasty meals that will make you feel like a rock star in the kitchen. I hope you grab this book on a regular basis and open it to your favorite quick recipe or try something new within these pages. With these recipes, you can lose weight, keep it off, and say goodbye to those awful diets for good, all while learning to enjoy delicious food again.

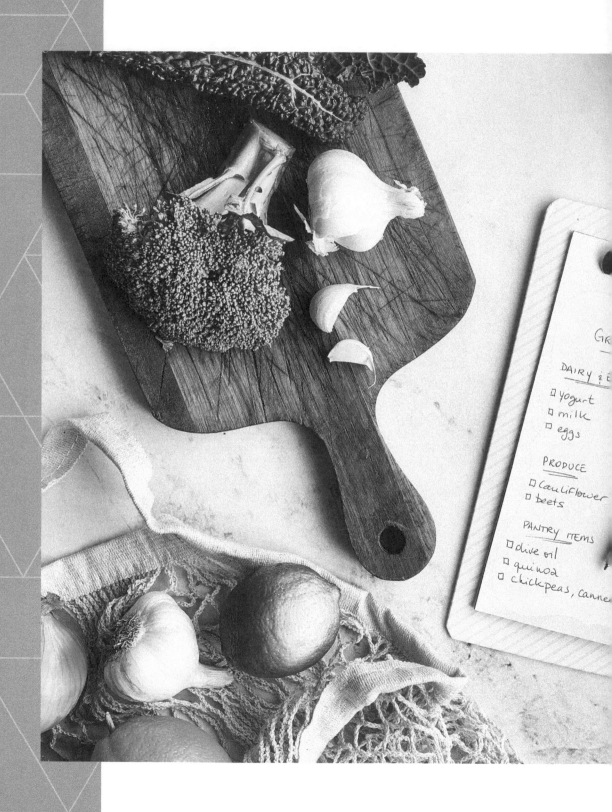

GR

DAIRY & E

☐ yogurt
☐ milk
☐ eggs

PRODUCE

☐ cauliflower
☐ beets

PANTRY ITEMS

☐ olive oil
☐ quinoa
☐ chickpeas, canne

CHAPTER ONE

Winning at Weight Loss

If you're done with diets, then you've come to the right place. "Diet" is a dirty four-letter word that overpromises and underdelivers. Quick, extreme weight-loss fixes consistently lead to frustration and failure. In fact, 95 percent of diets fail because they don't change habits for good—diets simply put bad habits on hold until you hit your goal or a wall.

While we all want to see immediate results, slow and steady wins the race when it comes to losing weight and keeping it off. This 30-minute meal approach to weight loss is an anti-diet. Rather than focusing on end results, this method focuses on the journey that leads to consistent, sustainable weight loss and, ultimately, maintenance of a healthy weight.

Along the way, you'll create delicious, healthy meals that aren't time-consuming or complicated. You'll acquire new tools and tricks to help you make the most of your time in the kitchen so you can move on with your day. And best of all, you'll find some new favorite recipes to keep adding to your meal plans because they're delicious and they fit into your lifestyle. We're all busy. Maintaining your weight and health shouldn't take over your life. Let's do it together, one 30-minute meal at a time.

DON'T LOSE YOURSELF IN LOSING WEIGHT

Most people associate weight loss with a number on the scale. If that's the focus for you, take a moment to reframe your perspective. Losing weight goes well beyond numbers. Weight loss is a feeling. It's having energy without relying on caffeine. Putting on that pair of jeans and strutting your stuff. Looking in the mirror and seeing your reflection smiling back. It's achieving a goal without realizing you even did it and not feeling deprived in the process.

You, my friend, are fabulous. If you came to this book initially for weight loss, great! But know that there's so much more than that for you here. There's support in your journey. Gone are the days of taking on weight loss on your own and hoping this time will be different. This time, I'll guide you along as you take a more caring, mindful approach that gets back to the reasons why we eat: for fuel and because food tastes good.

You may have seen this pattern before, known as the "diet cycle."

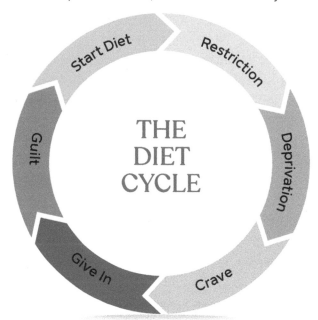

This diet cycle is the definition of insanity: doing the same thing over and over and expecting different results. Most diets don't work because they're unsustainable for the long haul. Diets typically require cutting out certain foods or even entire food groups. You may be told to put certain foods on your naughty list, which makes them even more desirable. Perhaps you've been told that if you just take this magic pill or drink a special shake, all your weight-loss problems will end. The thing is, if it were just as simple as just not eating a certain food or taking a pill or drinking a special potion, we wouldn't have an obesity epidemic that continues to rise in numbers. Those diets can leave you with a slower metabolism, risk of malnutrition, and an overall unhealthy relationship with food and your body.

I propose this: Instead of telling yourself everything you can't have, let's focus on the things you can do *more* of—things such as eating more fruits and vegetables, cooking easy and satisfying meals at home, and moving more in your day. You truly can do this with just a simple mindset reset.

But first, it's important to acknowledge that any weight-loss process is emotional, and that's okay. Hold space for yourself and your emotions throughout this book. Be kind to yourself. We're human and mistakes happen. Don't get hung up if something goes astray. There's no such thing as perfection. Learn from mistakes and high-five yourself on the small wins.

Before jumping into these recipes, take a moment to write down five things you love about yourself and your body that have nothing to do with weight. Perhaps it's those long legs that help you catch the subway. A scar with a great story behind it. Or your infectious smile. How does your body serve you well? Go ahead, write them down. I'll wait.

STARTING STRONG: CHANGE ONE HABIT

What is your *one* very worst food habit? It's okay—I'm not here to judge. Are you good about your eating habits all day but then binge at night? Does your barista have your afternoon mocha caramel latte waiting for you at the same time every day? Is dinner your only meal of the day?

Changing habits is a three-step process:

1. Become aware of the habits getting in your way.
2. Create a plan to change that habit.
3. Implement your plan with intention.

One of my favorite sayings is "small changes lead to big effects." I have personally seen this phenomenon over the years with my nutrition clients; simply making one small change leads to successful long-term outcomes.

The biggest pitfall I see in people trying to lead a healthier lifestyle occurs when they seek to make every possible change at once. Trying to change everything at once is overwhelming. If you want to see progress, choose one habit to change and focus on that.

Focusing on one habit allows you to stay on track and keep motivated. Perhaps instead of reaching for that daily 3:00 p.m. can of cola, you decide to swap it with a glass of water. That little change may not feel significant at first. But if each can is 140 calories, that's almost 1,000 calories a week and 4,000 calories a month. Keep in mind that 3,500 calories equals one pound. By simply swapping your daily cola with water, you can lose a pound in less than a month—just by making that one small change! Now you're motivated and wired to keep that habit while focusing on something new to change.

PHILOSOPHIES FOR WEIGHT MANAGEMENT

As a dietitian who promotes safe, healthy weight loss, I have a few simple philosophies for weight management:

All foods fit—there's no such thing as a "good" or "bad" food. The only foods you truly shouldn't eat are ones that have spoiled or dropped on the floor. Everything else is fair game. There are certainly foods you should consume and enjoy more often and others that are best to limit, but nothing is ever completely off the table. You have permission to eat foods that bring you joy. In this book, you will see recipes for carbs, desserts, and dishes that use butter as an ingredient. Ultimately, it all comes down to balance, variety, and portions.

Don't let numbers hold power over you. I have seen people make poor food choices because they're so fixated on hitting or staying under a certain number, such as total daily calories. For example, I've had clients choose 100-calorie packs of cookies because they think it's a better snack choice. The thing is, those calorie-controlled snack packs are not satisfying and often lead to eating multiple packs. An apple with peanut butter may be a 300-calorie snack, but it's more satisfying and curbs hunger for several hours. Paying more attention to what we're eating versus the numbers makes a tremendous difference in successful, long-term outcomes.

It all comes down to timing, quality, and quantity. First and foremost, don't skip meals. Eat every three to four hours for efficient metabolism, steady energy, and to keep hunger levels in check. Aim to consume quality wholesome foods with an emphasis on high-fiber foods, lean proteins, and healthy fats. Bring awareness to your portions. Use your plate as a guideline: Aim to fill half your plate with fruits and vegetables, one quarter with lean protein, and one quarter with healthy grains or starches.

OPTIMIZE YOUR RELATIONSHIP WITH FOOD

There are many reasons why we choose to lose weight. It could be for health or simply to feel good in your own skin. It's important to consider why you're making this choice. Mindfulness is a powerful tool that keeps us focused on *why* we eat versus *what* we eat. Here are three mindfulness exercises you can practice as you commit to following a healthy eating lifestyle:

THE HUNGER SCALE

On a 1 to 10 scale, where 1 is starving, 10 is Thanksgiving-dinner levels of fullness, and 5 is content, where does your hunger fall? If your stomach is growling and you rate hunger as a 3, then it's time for a meal or snack. But if you're just grabbing anything that's lying around, stop and check your hunger. If you determine your hunger level to be a 7, it probably means you're not actually hungry. Instead of eating, walk away and do something else to keep your mind occupied for a bit.

THE HUNGER SCALE

1	2	3	4	5	6	7	8	9	10
Starving, weak, dizzy	Very hungry, irritable, low energy, headache	Pretty hungry, stomach beginning to growl	Beginning to feel hungry	Comfortable, neither hungry nor full	Satisfied, but could eat more	Full and slightly uncomfortable	Stuffed and uncomfortably full	Very uncomfortable with stomachache	Painfully full, feeling sick

MAKE MEALTIME AN EXPERIENCE

Too often, we are distracted while eating, which leads to mindless overeating. To prevent this at mealtime, sit down at a table, plate your food, and put the distractions (including technology) away. Pay attention to what's happening on your plate. Do you have a good quality and quantity of foods? What colors do you see? How does it smell? Take the time to chew your food and really taste it. Savor your food and enjoy it. Engage in conversation between bites. It can take up to 20 minutes for your stomach to tell your brain it's full, so slow down to prevent overeating.

VISUALIZATION

Close your eyes. Imagine what life will look or feel like when you achieve and maintain weight loss. Write down three to five words associated with that visual and put it somewhere prominent. If you feel lost or frustrated, close your eyes, go back to your vision, and say those words out loud.

COOKING HACKS YOU NEED TO KNOW

We are all busy and our ultimate goal is to spend less time in the kitchen while still making delicious meals. These five kitchen hacks will help you become even more efficient in the kitchen.

1. **Read the recipe before you begin.** Nothing is worse than getting deep into a recipe and realizing you don't own the pan that's needed.

2. **Get out all tools and ingredients and line them up from left to right as listed in the recipe.** This is a major time-saver. And as my mom taught me, put the ingredient aside once you add it in case you forget if it was already used.

3. **Keep a trash can or scrap bowl nearby.** A handy trash can, large bowl, or plastic bag is great for trashing scraps as you're chopping up produce or meats and cuts down on time-wasting steps around the kitchen. Also, save food scraps to make broths and sauces and help reduce food waste.

4. **ABM—Always Be Multitasking.** While waiting for items to marinate, bake, or simmer, see what other steps can be completed in the preparation or cleaning process to cut down on time. This is another reason to read that recipe first.

5. **Use convenience cuts for the win.** Convenience cuts, or prewashed and precut fruits and vegetables, are available in a variety of options at the grocery store. Don't forget to check out frozen and canned produce options as well. They cut down on prep time and get meals on the table faster.

SHOPPING EFFICIENTLY

If you're trying to be efficient, never, ever set foot into a grocery store without a meal plan and a grocery list for putting the plan into action. This cuts down on time in the grocery store, saves money, reduces food waste, limits additional grocery store trips, and buys time during busy workweeks. I'm not a big proponent of only shopping the perimeter of the store, because the center aisles offer so many time-saving goodies. Make sure to visit these key grocery store sections:

Produce: Fresh fruits, veggies, and herbs

Deli, meats, and seafood: Fresh proteins, frozen seafood, and cooked rotisserie chickens

Grains and pastas: Fiber-rich sources of whole grains in dried and precooked forms

Cereal and snacks: Healthy breakfast and snack options like whole-grain cereals, nuts, popcorn, and crackers

Canned foods: Beans, tomatoes, veggies, fruits, broths, and seafood (look for low-sodium or no-added-salt options)

Baking ingredients: Flour, sugar, seasonings, and dried herbs

Condiments: Healthy cooking oils, dressings, marinades, and sauces

Dairy and eggs: More sources of protein to have alone or use as ingredients including milk, yogurt, and cheeses

Freezer: Frozen fruits and vegetables

Bakery: Fresh and packaged breads, English muffins, and tortillas

Bulk foods: If your store sells grains, dried beans, dried fruits, nuts, and seeds in bulk bins, these are a great way to try new items and only buy what you need.

Storage and household goods: Aluminum foil (regular and nonstick), parchment paper, wax paper, and zip-top bags

WHERE UNEXPECTED SABOTEURS HIDE

Food labels reveal key information about nutrients and ingredients in food. If you are unsure about a product, want to compare similar items, or are looking to add or reduce a certain nutrient, food labels give lots of helpful information.

For the whole story, read the entire label top to bottom. Pay special attention to serving sizes and how many servings are in the package. Read those labels with an open mind, and don't give yourself a calorie cut-off number without reviewing all the nutrients and ingredients.

Aim to keep saturated fat, trans fats, cholesterol, and sodium to a minimum. Don't let the total fat line item scare you. There are healthy sources of fats we want to consume, while keeping saturated fats to no more than 10 percent of total daily intake.

Don't fear the carbohydrate line item. Carbs are our main source of fuel and beneficial in adequate amounts. Aim to keep carbs between 15 and 30 grams per serving. More important is the amount of fiber in foods. Look for items that have a minimum of 3 grams of fiber per serving.

Limit added sugars. Dietary guidelines recommend under 50 grams total of daily added sources of sugars. Reading the ingredients list will help you determine the added sugars. Keep in mind that natural sweeteners, like honey, maple syrup, and fruit or vegetable juices, can show up as an added sugar, which is why reading the ingredient list is key. Sources of added sugars to limit include high fructose corn syrup, rice syrups, and various types of sugars. If a word ends in "-ose," that typically means it is some form of sugar.

Look for short ingredient lists. Overall, look for foods that contain minimal ingredients. Be mindful about front-of-label packaging, which can be deceiving in how nutrients are marketed. Instead, read the whole label, top to bottom, along with the ingredient list.

For a link to more info on how to read food labels, see the Resources section (page 158).

SET YOUR WORKSPACE UP FOR SUCCESS

A little planning and prep work can get meals on the table quickly. If you set everything up before you get started, you won't need to frequently move around your kitchen to get ingredients, tend to items on the stove, or scramble to pull out equipment. All those steps away from your workspace take time and reduce efficiency.

As a kitchen gadget lover, I'll admit I don't use those fabulous tools very often. They've just become something else I need to clean and put away, and since my goal is always to cut back on time in the kitchen, I opt for simpler tools. I've learned there is nothing a good-quality knife and cutting board can't do. I like kitchen tools and equipment that serve multiple functions. Read on for some of my must-have kitchen recommendations to help establish your own mega-efficient kitchen groove.

Essential Kitchen Tools

Baking dishes (2): Glass or stoneware dishes (9-by-13-inch and 8-by-8-inch) for baking and roasting.

Mixing and prep bowl set (1): A set of prep bowls in a variety of sizes, ranging from 1 ounce to 8 quarts, for prepping ingredients and mixing everything from seasonings to batters. Look for glass, microwave-safe options.

Nonstick skillets (3): I recommend 8-, 10-, and 13-inch oven-safe skillets with nonstick surfaces for easy cleanup. The largest one should come with a lid for quick cooking and keeping food warm.

Pots (3): A 6-quart stockpot is perfect for making soups, sauces, and one-pot meals. Many also come with a handy steamer attachment. You'll also want 1- and 3-quart pots with lids for sauces, grains, and pastas.

Sheet pans (2): Sheet pans, also known as baking sheets, are typically 13 by 18 inches. Look for options that include a cooling rack, which helps create crispy textures. Since I encourage using nonstick foil or parchment paper to minimize cleanup, standard aluminum pans are perfect.

Slow at Prep? There's a Gadget for That!

Citrus press: Marinades, dressings, and sauces often call for citrus juice. Fresh citrus has greater nutritional quality and flavor than bottled varieties, so using a press will quickly add juices directly into recipes.

Cookie scoops: A cookie scoop saves a ton of time and ensures that each cookie, meatball, or muffin comes out evenly sized. Get a set of 1-, 2-, and 3-tablespoon scoops.

Food processor: Although they make mini versions that only chop, I recommend a standard version with chopping, grating, and slicing attachments for optimum convenience.

Immersion blender with attachments: I admitted I'm not a big gadget user, but this is one of my top-used items in the kitchen. Look for immersion blenders that come with a chopping and whisk attachment to cover many prep needs.

Knife set: Quality knives make prep work fast and easy. The most important knives to have are a chef's knife and paring knife. Ideal sets also include kitchen shears, great for chopping herbs, and a sharpener for keeping blades sharp and efficient.

TIME-SAVING INGREDIENTS

There will come a day when you can't get to the store or your plans fall through and now you're cooking instead of going out. If you stock your pantry, refrigerator, and freezer with key ingredients, you'll be covered and ready to prepare healthy, home-cooked meals on the spot.

I'm all about a good shortcut when it comes to meal preparation. Grocery stores and food companies recognize that people are busy and are offering more healthy convenience options than ever before. If you don't already have the following items in your kitchen, now's the time to stock up so you can start using them to create 30-minute meals.

Pantry

Canned beans: Canned beans and legumes add plant-based proteins to salads, bowls, and soups. Keep a variety on hand, including chickpeas and black, kidney, and cannellini beans.

Canned/dried fruits and vegetables: Shelf-stable fruits and vegetables can be just as nutritious as fresh. Keep canned fruits like pineapple, peaches, pears, and mandarin oranges available to toss into recipes or create marinades and sauces. Dried fruits such as raisins, figs, and dates add sweetness and fiber to dishes. Vegetables, including artichoke hearts, sun-dried tomatoes, and roasted red peppers, can enhance meals quickly and easily.

Canned tomatoes: Whole, sauce, crushed, diced, or paste, canned tomatoes are a must-have staple. Canned tomatoes add texture to sauces, soups, and side dishes.

Canned tuna and salmon: A handy shelf-stable source of protein, canned (or packets of) seafood can be added to salads and pasta dishes, as well as formed into patties.

Dried herbs and spices: Stock your pantry with spices like basil, oregano, cumin, and chili powder—there's no easier way to add flavor to a meal. Look for seasoning blends as well, such as Italian or everything bagel.

Whole grains and pastas: Grains and pastas can be high-fiber sources of carbohydrates. Whole grains include quinoa, oats, and barley, to name a few. Pasta can also be part of a healthy lifestyle; just look for options that have at least 2 to 3 grams of fiber. Some pastas are made from chickpeas, lentils, and black beans—these add protein to meals.

Refrigerator

Cheese: Grated Parmesan, fresh mozzarella, shredded cheeses, and sliced cheese are versatile and add flavor to many recipes. Keep a variety on hand to use as ingredients or toppers.

Eggs: Whether eggs are the star or a supporting cast member, they fit into countless meals and recipes. Hard-boiled eggs are also available for purchase and can make a quick protein addition to meals.

Fresh fruits and vegetables: Look for convenient prewashed and cut options, such as mango, pineapple, broccoli and cauliflower florets, and sliced mushrooms. Prewashed leafy greens are ready to go for salads or sauté for sides. Carrots, celery, and onions add flavor and nutrition as a base in soups and sauces.

Greek yogurt: Swap out high-calorie ingredients like sour cream and mayo with Greek yogurt for added protein and less saturated fat. It's also perfect for sauces and dressings.

Herbs: Fresh herbs elevate the flavor of meals. Keep fresh herbs like basil, thyme, rosemary, parsley, and cilantro on hand. I prefer to purchase the smaller prepped containers of herbs versus the bunches if I just need a little.

Milk: Whether you choose dairy or plant-based milk, this staple adds creaminess and liquid to recipes. Choose low-fat or nonfat options.

Freezer

Frozen fruits: Frozen fruits such as berries, mango, and açai can make quick smoothies, desserts, and even sauces.

Frozen herbs, garlic, and ginger: Did you know you can purchase herbs, garlic, and ginger in convenient, preportioned frozen form? Thaw in the microwave for recipes that require fresh options, or toss into stovetop dishes right from the freezer.

Frozen pasta: Frozen gnocchi and ravioli make quick meals. In addition to traditional potato gnocchi and cheese ravioli, look for varieties stuffed with cauliflower, spinach, artichoke, and sweet potato.

Frozen seafood: Unlike many proteins, frozen seafood can usually be thawed quickly. Frozen shrimp cooks up nicely straight from the freezer.

Frozen vegetables: Whether you choose to steam, sauté, or roast, frozen veggies are one of my favorite time-saving staples. At the top of the list is frozen chopped onions. So many recipes call for chopped onions, and these are a lifesaver in a pinch.

Frozen veggie burgers: Frozen veggie and black bean burgers add plant-based protein to salads, bowls, and wraps. You can even crumble them up for tacos. Try swapping them for some protein options shared in this book.

OPTIMIZE YOUR INGREDIENTS

As you can see, this book aims to save you as much time as possible in the kitchen, even before you start cooking. To save even more time, use these tips to extend the life of your foods and make fewer trips to the store.

- Most fresh fruits and vegetables can be frozen as long as they have a low water content (not watermelon, cucumbers, or iceberg lettuce).
- Organic milk lasts longer than regular milk.
- Once an avocado ripens, put it in the refrigerator to slow the ripening process.
- Freeze fresh herbs in ice cube trays with water or olive oil, then add to sautés, sauces, or soups as needed.
- Don't store potatoes and onions near each other, as they will cause each other to spoil.
- Store nuts in the freezer to prevent the oils from becoming rancid.
- Store unpeeled garlic cloves in an airtight container in the refrigerator.
- Stand fresh herbs, asparagus, and scallions in a glass partially filled with water in the refrigerator.
- Don't store tomatoes, bananas, or potatoes in the refrigerator, as they will become mushy.
- Store honey at room temperature, and refrigerate pure maple syrup.

TAME YOUR CLEANUP TIME

Nobody likes cleaning up, especially when you're trying to spend less time in the kitchen. The following cleanup hacks can ensure that you sit down for meals without a major mess to tackle afterward.

Use zip-top bags for seasoning and marinating. Gallon-size zip-top bags are great for marinating and mixing ingredients together to cut down on bowls to wash. Place your ingredients in a bag, add your seasonings or marinade, remove the air, seal, and shake or massage. Discard the used bag.

Focus on sheet pan, one-pot, and foil packet meals. You'll see recipes like these throughout this book, and the more of these meals you have in your repertoire, the less cleanup you'll have in your life.

Make nonstick aluminum foil and parchment paper your cleanup BFFs. No one has time to fight with baked-on cheese, so get in the habit of lining pans and dishes for easy cleanup. You can also spray regular foil with nonstick cooking spray.

Soak dishes while eating. Place dirty dishes and pans in hot soapy water while you eat to soften them for easier scrubbing later.

Clean as you go. Remember ABM (Always Be Multitasking, see page 7)? Tidy your workspace as you go or while items cook. This will prevent one big mess to deal with after a delicious dinner.

TIME SAVED = TIME EARNED

You know what's the best part about getting meals on the table in under 30 minutes? All the time you gain back in your life! Time is often the biggest reason that I hear from people for why they don't exercise or practice self-care.

Weight management is about more than just the quality and quantity of food you eat. It's about moving your body, staying hydrated, managing stress, and getting a good night's sleep. Your body requires 360 degrees of holistic care. So give yourself and your body some love, will ya?

Once you're mastering those quick meals, I have a challenge for you: What are some ways you can do something for *you* in your day with that extra time? Here are a few ideas to get you going:

▶ Take a walk around the block.

▶ Run up and down the stairs a few times.

▶ Rep out some squats or see how long you can hold a plank while waiting for items to bake.

▶ Do a short high-intensity workout.

▶ Grab your partner and dance.

▶ Enjoy a big glass of water or a warm cup of tea.

▶ Take three deep, mindful breaths.

▶ Listen to a meditation podcast or app.

▶ Take a bubble bath.

▶ Do a facial mask.

▶ Unplug from social media and electronics just to be in the moment.

▶ Go to bed earlier than usual and get a good night's sleep.

I'm so excited for you and grateful to be part of your journey. Now, let's get into the real reason you're here: the recipes!

ABOUT THE RECIPES

You already know the recipes in this book are easy and can all be done in 30 minutes. I'm sure it's a big part of what attracted you to this book in the first place. But let's discuss the facets of "easy" that are baked into each recipe.

Labels that indicate special features. Many of these recipes fall into the following categories:
- One-Pot (uses one main piece of equipment, such as a skillet or sheet pan)
- 5-Ingredient (excludes nonstick cooking spray, oil, water, salt, and black pepper)
- Extra Low Calorie (400 calories or less)
  These recipes will be labeled as such, and you can also reference them in the Index.

Tips that make the recipe even easier. All recipes will feature one of the following pro tips:
- Simple Swap (such as using dried herbs if fresh isn't available)
- Cooking Hack (like using a microwave to cook vegetables—yes, even the pros do it)
- Technique Trick (like how to make carrot ribbons for your salad)
- Love Your Leftovers (how to repurpose your leftovers)
- Serving Suggestion (such as side dish suggestions)

Store-bought suggestions. To keep the recipes in the 30-minute time frame, I'll recommend ready-to-use store-bought ingredients when appropriate. Look for minimally processed ingredients to add to your meals—this is where reading food labels comes in handy.

Use your plate for portion control. While I don't encourage counting calories or using food scales, I do encourage you to take notice of what is happening at meals and showing up on your plate. A big part of mindful eating is awareness of the quality and quantity of foods you are enjoying at meals and snacks. MyPlate (page 158) is a tool I have used with clients for years that emphasizes eating for wellness.
Use your plate as a guideline for how to plan and portion meals:
- Fill half the plate with fruits and veggies. These are the best bang for your nutritional buck, loaded with satisfying fiber to curb hunger. Try for two palm-size servings of vegetables, a palm-size serving each of veggies and fruit, or a palm- or fist-size serving of fruit.

- Fill one quarter of the plate with your lean protein source. Aim for no larger than the palm of your hand.
- Fill the final quarter with starches or grains. This can include starchy vegetables, such as potatoes, winter squash, or corn, as well as whole grains, rice, pasta, breads, or beans. This should also be kept to the size of your palm or fist for portion control. Emphasize high-fiber options when possible.

I chose to share the following recipes with the hope that you'll keep coming back to these meals because they're easy and tasty. Perhaps you'll have a few on regular rotation, and I always encourage you to try new ones along the way. I hope these recipes introduce you to some new foods and ingredients, provide new twists on your favorites, rekindle your love of some food items you thought you had to break up with in order to manage your weight, and teach you some time-saving tips and tricks along the way. Now, let's get cooking!

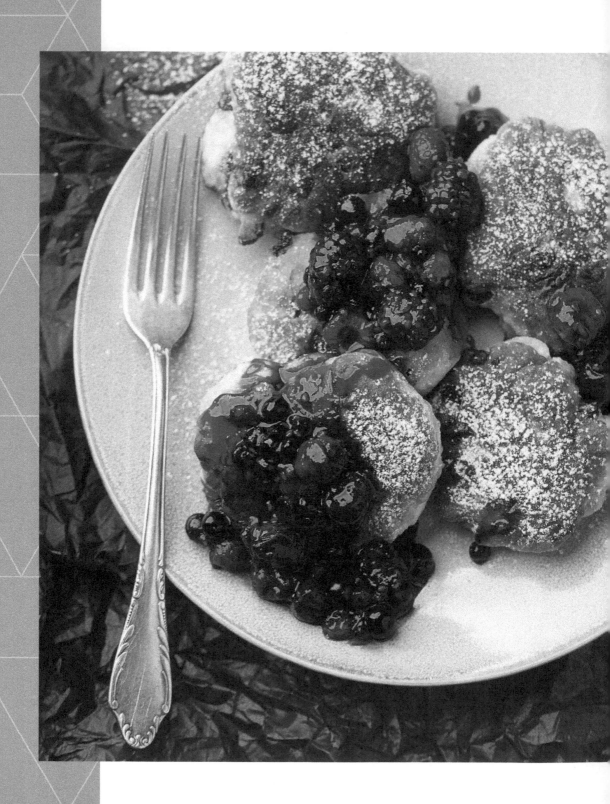

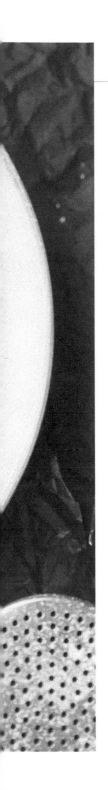

Breakfast

Welcome to the most important meal of the day! If you tend to skip breakfast, I urge you to reconsider. Breakfast has been shown to help with weight loss and weight management because it helps kick-start your metabolism for the day, keep hunger levels in check, and maintain energy levels. These breakfast recipes provide a variety of sweet, savory, and hearty flavors while keeping your weight in check. Oh, and don't be fooled by the word "breakfast"—I'm a huge brinner (breakfast for dinner) fan. Many of these meals can be your last of the day as well as your first.

CHOCOLATE-ZUCCHINI SMOOTHIE

EXTRA LOW CALORIE   ONE-POT
PREP TIME: 5 minutes
SERVES 1

Enjoy the flavor of zucchini bread without the effort of baking. This smoothie blends together fresh zucchini with a mix of superfoods including cacao, walnuts, oats, and flaxseed. Loaded with antioxidants, this smoothie will help keep cells healthy and fight inflammation, also benefitting weight management.

½ cup nonfat milk (or non-dairy alternative)

½ zucchini, coarsely chopped

½ frozen banana

1 tablespoon cacao powder

1 teaspoon cacao nibs

2 tablespoons walnuts

1 teaspoon maple syrup

1 tablespoon rolled oats

1 tablespoon ground flaxseed

¼ cup plain nonfat Greek yogurt

1. Pour the milk into a blender. Add the zucchini, banana, cacao powder, cacao nibs, walnuts, maple syrup, rolled oats, flaxseed, and yogurt.

2. Blend for 30 to 60 seconds, or to your desired consistency. Use additional milk to thin, if desired.

SIMPLE SWAP: If you don't have cacao powder or nibs, swap them with 1 tablespoon cocoa powder or dark chocolate chips.

PER SERVING: Calories: 334; Total fat: 15g; Saturated fat: 2g; Sodium: 97mg; Carbohydrates: 41g; Fiber: 8g; Protein: 17g; Calcium: 281mg; Potassium: 1,052mg

GOLDEN MILK SMOOTHIE

EXTRA LOW CALORIE   ONE-POT
PREP TIME: 5 minutes
SERVES 1

Golden milk, traditionally served as a warm beverage, gets its golden color from turmeric. Turmeric, as well as ginger and cinnamon, are loaded with antioxidants that keep cells healthy, boost immunity, and promote digestion, which plays a key role in weight management. Kefir is a drinkable form of yogurt called the "Champagne of Dairy" for its effervescence. It is a powerful probiotic that's also great for digestive health.

¼ cup nonfat milk

1 cup frozen mango

½ frozen banana

¾ cup plain kefir

1 teaspoon honey

1 teaspoon ground turmeric

½ teaspoon ground cinnamon

1 teaspoon ground flaxseed

¼ teaspoon ground ginger

Pinch cayenne or freshly ground black pepper (optional)

1. Pour the milk into a blender. Add the mango, banana, kefir, honey, turmeric, cinnamon, flaxseed, ginger, and cayenne (if using).

2. Blend for 30 to 60 seconds, or to your desired consistency.

COOKING HACK: As fresh bananas ripen, slice them and place into small freezer-safe bags for use in recipes like smoothies. You can also blend fresh banana with ice for a creamy consistency.

PER SERVING: Calories: 296; Total fat: 6g; Saturated fat: 3g; Sodium: 86mg; Carbohydrates: 56g; Fiber: 6g; Protein: 9g; Calcium: 270mg; Potassium: 873mg

AÇAI SMOOTHIE BOWL

ONE-POT

PREP TIME: 10 minutes

SERVES 1 OR 2

Just because a smoothie bowl is made with fruit doesn't automatically make it a healthy option. Some smoothie bowls have as many calories as an ice cream sundae! This better-for-you option cuts back on the added sweeteners and juices while pumping in protein and fiber. The addition of frozen cauliflower provides a creamy texture like frozen bananas without the extra carbs. The trick to a good smoothie bowl? A high-speed blender and all frozen fruit.

1 frozen açai packet

½ cup frozen mixed berries

½ frozen banana

½ cup frozen cauliflower florets

¾ cup plain nonfat Greek yogurt

1 tablespoon hemp seeds

1 tablespoon chia seeds

2 tablespoons rolled oats

1 tablespoon nut or seed butter

¼ cup unsweetened almond milk

Granola, nuts, seeds, and/or fruit, for topping (optional)

1. Run the frozen açai packet under hot water for 5 seconds to soften. Do not defrost.

2. In a high-speed blender, combine the açai, berries, banana, cauliflower, yogurt, hemp seeds, chia seeds, rolled oats, nut butter, and almond milk.

3. Blend for 1 to 3 minutes at medium-high speed, stopping every 15 seconds to push down the ingredients with a tamper or rubber spatula for even blending.

4. Blend to your desired consistency. If too thin, add 1 cup of ice to the blender. If too thick, add additional milk, ¼ cup at a time.

5. Pour the mixture into a bowl and top with add-ons of choice, such as granola, nuts, seeds, or additional fruit.

COOKING HACK: If you don't own a high-speed blender, a food processor with a puree setting can create equally creamy smoothie bowls. Pulse a few times, scrape down the sides, and repeat until you reach your desired consistency.

PER SERVING (FULL RECIPE): Calories: 514; Total fat: 21g; Saturated fat: 3g; Sodium: 139mg; Carbohydrates: 58g; Fiber: 15g; Protein: 28g; Calcium: 452mg; Potassium: 978mg

BAKED OATMEAL CUPS

EXTRA LOW CALORIE

PREP TIME: 10 minutes   **COOK TIME:** 20 minutes

SERVES 6

What's better than a quick breakfast? A breakfast you can enjoy even faster for the rest of the week! I love making a batch of these oatmeal cups on the weekend and eating them throughout the week. Enjoy them on their own, or top them with yogurt and additional fruit, nuts, and seeds for a fiber-filled breakfast or snack option that's more satisfying than a traditional muffin.

Nonstick cooking spray (optional)

2 cups rolled oats

1 teaspoon baking powder

1 teaspoon ground cinnamon, plus more for garnish if desired

¼ teaspoon kosher salt

1 cup nonfat milk

2 large eggs

¼ cup maple syrup

¼ cup unsweetened applesauce

1 teaspoon vanilla extract

½ cup dried cranberries

½ cup pecan halves

1. Preheat the oven to 350ºF. Line a 12-cup muffin tin with paper liners or use cooking spray.

2. In a medium bowl, stir together the oats, baking powder, cinnamon, and salt.

3. Add the milk, eggs, maple syrup, applesauce, and vanilla. Stir to combine until well mixed. Fold in the cranberries and pecans.

4. Using a ¼-cup measuring scoop, divide the batter evenly into the muffin cups. Sprinkle each oatmeal cup with cinnamon, if desired. Bake for 20 minutes, until they are golden brown on the top and a toothpick inserted into the center comes out clean. Allow to cool for a few minutes.

5. Store leftover oatmeal cups in a sealed container at room temperature for up to 5 days or freeze for up to 3 months. If desired, warm in a microwave on high for 1 minute or in a 350ºF oven for 3 to 5 minutes.

SIMPLE SWAP: Try different nut and fruit combos, such as blueberries and almonds or raisins and walnuts.

PER SERVING: Calories: 293; Total fat: 10g; Saturated fat: 1g; Sodium: 95mg; Carbohydrates: 44g; Fiber: 5g; Protein: 8g; Calcium: 132mg; Potassium: 347mg

SAVORY PESTO OATS

5-INGREDIENT   EXTRA LOW CALORIE
PREP TIME: 5 minutes   COOK TIME: 5 minutes
SERVES 2

Savory oatmeal changes up breakfast and makes a perfect option for those who don't like sweet meals. Cooking oats in broth and mixing in a sauce like pesto gives oatmeal flavors you didn't know it could have. Top with an egg for added protein. The best part? This dish comes together super fast!

Nonstick cooking spray

1 cup rolled oats

1¾ cups chicken or vegetable broth

2 tablespoons Spinach-Pistachio Pesto Sauce (page 140) or any store-bought pesto

2 tablespoons shredded part-skim mozzarella cheese, plus more for garnish

2 large eggs

Red pepper flakes, for garnish (optional)

1. Spray a nonstick skillet over medium heat with cooking spray.

2. In a microwave-safe bowl, stir together the oats and broth. Microwave on high for 3 minutes.

3. Remove from the microwave and stir in the pesto and mozzarella cheese. Divide into two bowls.

4. While the oatmeal is in the microwave, prepare the eggs to your preference (over easy or sunny-side up work well). Place a cooked egg on top of each bowl of oats. Garnish with additional mozzarella and red pepper flakes (if using).

SIMPLE SWAP: Create a Southwestern version by using ¼ cup salsa in place of the pesto and cheddar cheese instead of mozzarella. Top with your favorite hot sauce.

PER SERVING: Calories: 378; Total fat: 18g; Saturated fat: 5g; Sodium: 451mg; Carbohydrates: 35g; Fiber: 5g; Protein: 17g; Calcium: 147mg; Potassium: 300mg

SPINACH AND CHEDDAR ALMOST EGGS BENEDICT

5-INGREDIENT

PREP TIME: 5 minutes **COOK TIME:** 5 minutes

SERVES 2

I was inspired by a local beachfront restaurant near my home at the Jersey Shore that makes a version of this dish. It always reminds me of summer. I call it an "almost" Benedict because I am terrible at poaching eggs and found that over easy–style works just as well to provide that runny yolk goodness. This version uses melted cheese in place of high-fat hollandaise sauce and spinach in place of Canadian bacon.

2 whole-grain English muffins, split

2 tablespoons olive oil, divided

6 cups fresh baby spinach

4 large eggs

4 slices deli cheddar cheese, such as Vermont cheddar

Salt

Freshly ground black pepper

1. Lightly toast the English muffins and divide between two plates.

2. In a large nonstick skillet, heat 1 tablespoon of oil over medium heat. Add the spinach and sauté until it just starts to wilt, 2 to 3 minutes.

3. Remove the spinach from the skillet and divide it evenly on top of the English muffins.

4. In the same skillet, heat the remaining 1 tablespoon of oil and crack the eggs into it. Allow to cook for 1 minute, until the bottoms are slightly browned and yolks are set. Turn the heat to low, flip the eggs, and top each egg with a slice of cheese. Cover the pan and cook for 1 minute, until the cheese is melted. The yolks will be slightly runny. If you prefer a harder yolk, cook for an additional 1 to 2 minutes.

5. Uncover and remove the skillet from the heat. Place the eggs with cheese over the spinach-topped English muffins. Season with salt and pepper and enjoy immediately.

SIMPLE SWAP: Frozen spinach can be used in place of fresh spinach and can either be sautéed in the pan or microwaved with 1 to 2 tablespoons vegetable broth to add flavor. Reduce the amount to 4 cups if using frozen spinach.

PER SERVING: Calories: 644; Total fat: 44g; Saturated fat: 16g; Sodium: 892mg; Carbohydrates: 31g; Fiber: 6g; Protein: 34g; Calcium: 698mg; Potassium: 822mg

BAKED VEGETABLE FRITTATA

5-INGREDIENT　EXTRA LOW CALORIE　ONE-POT
PREP TIME: 5 minutes　**COOK TIME:** 25 minutes
SERVES 6

One of the biggest complaints I hear is that eggs are too hard to make during the week. I challenge that statement! This baked frittata takes just minutes to put together and can bake while you get ready for work. Any combination of veggies works, making it a great way to use up leftovers or produce starting to go south. Use a muffin tin instead of a baking dish for individual portions. Serve with mixed greens or fruits for a complete meal.

Nonstick cooking spray

8 large eggs

2 tablespoons nonfat milk

Salt

Freshly ground black pepper

1 cup baby spinach, packed

¼ cup grape tomatoes, halved

¼ cup shredded cheddar cheese or other cheese of choice, plus more for topping if desired

1. Preheat the oven to 400°F. Spray an 8-by-8-inch baking dish with cooking spray.

2. In a medium bowl, whisk together the eggs and milk, then season with salt and pepper. Stir in the spinach, tomatoes, and cheese.

3. Pour the mixture into the prepared baking pan. Top with an additional sprinkle of cheese if desired. Bake for 20 minutes, or until the middle is set. Allow to cool for 5 minutes, then slice into six squares.

4. Store leftovers in the refrigerator for up to 4 days, and reheat in the microwave on high for 1 minute.

COOKING HACK: Make cleanup even easier by lining the baking dish with a piece of parchment paper cut to fit the bottom of the pan.

PER SERVING: Calories: 118; Total fat: 8g; Saturated fat: 3g; Sodium: 157mg; Carbohydrates: 1g; Fiber: 1g; Protein: 10g; Calcium: 81mg; Potassium: 146mg

SHEET PAN VEGGIE HASH

EXTRA LOW CALORIE   ONE-POT

PREP TIME: 5 minutes   **COOK TIME:** 25 minutes

SERVES 6

Start your day with a low-carb hash loaded with roasted veggies and eggs, cooked on the same pan for a relaxing breakfast with minimal cleanup. The more precut veggies you can buy ahead of time, the faster this hash will come together. This dish also makes a fantastic dinner option.

2 cups chopped fresh or frozen broccoli florets

2 cups sliced mushrooms

1 cup diced red onion

1 cup diced red bell pepper

1 cup grape tomatoes, halved

2 tablespoons olive oil

1 teaspoon dried thyme

Salt

Freshly ground black pepper

6 large eggs

½ cup shredded cheddar Jack cheese

1. Preheat the oven to 425°F. Line a sheet pan with nonstick aluminum foil.

2. In a large bowl, combine the broccoli, mushrooms, onion, bell pepper, and tomatoes. Add the olive oil and thyme and season with salt and pepper. Stir to coat the vegetables.

3. Spread the vegetables in a single layer on the sheet pan. Bake on the center oven rack for 15 minutes.

4. Remove the pan from the oven. Using the back of a serving spoon, create 6 wells in the hash. Crack an egg into a small cup or bowl, then pour into one of the wells. Repeat with the remaining eggs. Sprinkle the shredded cheese over the hash.

5. Return the pan to the oven and cook for an additional 6 to 10 minutes, or until the egg whites are cooked through and solid. If you prefer runny eggs, cook them less; for harder yolks, cook longer. The eggs will continue to cook once removed from the oven. Serve immediately.

6. Store leftover hash in the refrigerator for up to 4 days.

LOVE YOUR LEFTOVERS: Don't cook all the eggs if you plan on saving any leftover hash. Reheat the leftovers in the oven or toaster oven at 425°F for 5 minutes, or until the veggies are warmed. Cook the eggs as directed. Top with additional cheese.

PER SERVING: Calories: 188; Total fat: 13g; Saturated fat: 2g; Sodium: 172mg; Carbohydrates: 8g; Fiber: 4g; Protein: 11g; Calcium: 117mg; Potassium: 397mg

MUSHROOM, KALE, AND FETA BREAKFAST TACOS WITH BRUSCHETTA TOPPING

EXTRA LOW CALORIE
PREP TIME: 5 minutes   **COOK TIME:** 15 minutes
SERVES 3

Move over tacos with eggs and salsa—these breakfast tacos get a Mediterranean makeover with veggies, feta, and a bruschetta topping. They come together in no time, thanks to the help of store-bought and prepped ingredients. Prechopped kale, sliced mushrooms, and ready-made tomato bruschetta make this satisfying breakfast a perfect post-workout refuel.

1 tablespoon avocado oil

1 cup sliced mushrooms

4 large eggs

1 tablespoon nonfat milk

¼ teaspoon dried basil

⅛ teaspoon freshly ground black pepper

1 cup chopped kale

Nonstick cooking spray (optional)

¼ cup crumbled feta cheese

6 (6-inch) corn tortillas

1 cup prepared tomato bruschetta topping

1. In a 10-inch skillet, heat the oil over medium heat.

2. Add the mushrooms and sauté for 2 to 3 minutes, until softened, stirring often.

3. In a small bowl, whisk together the eggs, milk, basil, and pepper and set aside.

4. Add the kale to the skillet and sauté for 1 minute, until wilted.

5. If needed, spray the skillet with cooking spray before adding the egg mixture to the skillet. Using a spatula, scramble together the eggs with the vegetables. As the eggs set, stir in the feta crumbles and sauté for another minute, until the cheese is softened.

6. Assemble the tacos by dividing the egg mixture among the tortillas, and top each with bruschetta topping.

COOKING HACK: Warm the tortillas in a nonstick 8-inch skillet over high heat by placing them individually on each side for 10 seconds. Alternatively, wrap the stack of tortillas in a paper towel and microwave them on high for 1 minute.

PER SERVING: Calories: 293; Total fat: 15g; Saturated fat: 5g; Sodium: 239mg; Carbohydrates: 26g; Fiber: 4g; Protein: 15g; Calcium: 159mg; Potassium: 417mg

TURKEY SAUSAGE BREAKFAST SANDWICHES

PREP TIME: 10 minutes   **COOK TIME:** 15 minutes
SERVES 6

With lean ground turkey and seasonings, you can create sausage patties that are lower in saturated fat, sodium, and calories than store-bought varieties. Make a batch of these patties to reheat during the week. Extra patties are a great way to add protein to pasta dishes, like Penne Vodka with Artichokes and Roasted Red Peppers (page 71).

1 pound ground turkey

1 teaspoon dried fennel

1 teaspoon ground sage

½ teaspoon onion powder

½ teaspoon garlic powder

½ teaspoon dried parsley

¼ teaspoon sea salt

⅛ teaspoon freshly ground black pepper

1 tablespoon olive oil

6 whole-wheat English muffins, split

6 Granny Smith apple slices, ¼ inch thick

6 slices deli cheddar cheese

1. In a large bowl, combine the ground turkey, fennel, sage, onion powder, garlic powder, parsley, salt, and pepper. Using your hands, combine the ingredients until well blended.

2. Shape the turkey into six patties, about 3 inches in diameter.

3. Preheat the oven broiler on high.

4. In a large oven-safe skillet, heat the olive oil over medium heat. Cook the sausage patties for 5 minutes on each side, until cooked through (internal temperature of 165°F).

5. Toast the English muffins in the toaster.

6. When the patties are done, remove them from the heat and top each with one apple slice and one slice of cheddar. Place the pan under the broiler for 60 to 90 seconds, until the cheese is melted.

7. Place each patty on an English muffin half. Top with the other half. Serve immediately.

8. Store leftover patties in the refrigerator for 3 to 4 days or freeze for up to 3 months.

LOVE YOUR LEFTOVERS: If you don't plan to make all the sandwiches, cook the sausage patties up through step 4. Cool before transferring to the refrigerator. Reheat patties as needed throughout the week to assemble sandwiches with the apple and cheddar.

PER SERVING: Calories: 465; Total fat: 19g; Saturated fat: 7g; Sodium: 563mg; Carbohydrates: 47g; Fiber: 9g; Protein: 28g; Calcium: 389mg; Potassium: 519mg

CHICKEN CHORIZO AND EGG
BREAKFAST SKILLET

ONE-POT

PREP TIME: 5 minutes   **COOK TIME:** 10 minutes

SERVES **4**

Nothing is easier in the morning than tossing everything into a skillet. This dish is a great way to get protein from eggs along with fiber-rich vegetables in the morning. Using chicken chorizo in place of traditional pork chorizo cuts down on calories and saturated fat. Any leftovers make for a quick and easy breakfast to reheat during a busy workweek.

2 tablespoons avocado oil, divided

2 chicken chorizo sausage links, diced

1 jalapeño, seeds removed and diced (optional)

6 large eggs

¼ cup scallions, sliced

2 tablespoons nonfat milk

1 (10-ounce) can fire roasted diced tomatoes with green chiles, drained (or plain diced tomatoes)

½ cup shredded four-cheese Mexican blend

1 avocado, peeled, pitted, and diced

1. In a 10-inch nonstick skillet, heat 1 tablespoon of oil over medium heat.

2. Add the chorizo and jalapeño (if using), sautéing until the chorizo is browned and the jalapeño is tender, 5 minutes.

3. In a small bowl, whisk together the eggs, scallions, and milk and set aside.

4. When the chorizo and jalapeño mixture is ready, stir in the diced tomatoes with chiles until combined. Add the remaining 1 tablespoon of oil and the egg mixture.

5. Use a rubber spatula to scramble the eggs by pushing the mixture to the side of the pan until curds start to form. As the eggs become solid, stir in the cheese until melted and combined. Remove from the heat and top with diced avocado. Serve immediately.

6. Store leftovers in the refrigerator for up to 4 days.

SERVING SUGGESTION: Enjoy this skillet on its own as a low-carb option or serve with tortillas or Jalapeño-Cheddar Corn Muffins (page 62).

PER SERVING: Calories: 442; Total fat: 35g; Saturated fat: 10g; Sodium: 678mg; Carbohydrates: 9g; Fiber: 5g; Protein: 22g; Calcium: 183mg; Potassium: 593mg

SWEET POTATO TOAST WITH ALMOND BUTTER AND BANANA

EXTRA LOW CALORIE   ONE-POT
PREP TIME: 5 minutes   **COOK TIME:** 15 minutes
SERVES 4

Who says bread gets to have all the fun when it comes to toast? Put slices of sweet potato in the toaster to heat, crisp, and top—you'll boost your veggies with this fun and easy breakfast option. This version uses almond butter, banana slices, seeds, and honey for some sweetness, but you can get creative and decorate your sweet potato toast any way you'd like. Try avocado, cottage cheese, or an egg!

1 large (or 2 medium) sweet potatoes, unpeeled, cut diagonally into ¼-inch slices

Nonstick cooking spray

2 tablespoons almond butter (or any nut or seed butter)

1 banana, sliced

Hemp seeds, for garnish

Cinnamon, for garnish

Honey, for garnish

1. Spray both sides of the sweet potato slices with cooking spray. Place the slices directly on the rack of a toaster oven and toast on the highest setting. Repeat toasting until the sweet potato slices are browned and toasted on the outside, cooked through, and somewhat crisp. This may take 2 or 3 rounds, approximately 5 minutes per round. If you use a pop-up toaster, the cooking time may take a little longer.

2. Spread the almond butter on the potato slices and top with a few banana slices. Garnish with hemp seeds, cinnamon, and a drizzle of honey.

COOKING HACK: A mandoline can create thinner slices of potato so they cook even faster.

PER SERVING: Calories: 109; Total fat: 5g; Saturated fat: 0g; Sodium: 19mg; Carbohydrates: 15g; Fiber: 3g; Protein: 3g; Calcium: 39mg; Potassium: 275mg

BUCKWHEAT PANCAKES WITH BERRY COMPOTE

EXTRA LOW CALORIE

PREP TIME: 5 minutes   **COOK TIME:** 25 minutes

SERVES 4

Nothing says the weekend better than pancakes. Buckwheat boosts the fiber and protein content of traditional pancakes for a hearty and satisfying meal. This uses berry compote in place of syrup for a sweet topping.

2 cups frozen mixed berries

2 tablespoons pomegranate juice

¾ cup buckwheat flour

¾ cup self-rising flour (see Simple Swap)

1 tablespoon sugar

¼ teaspoon baking soda

½ teaspoon ground cinnamon

2 teaspoons chia seeds, divided

2 large eggs

1 cup buttermilk

1 teaspoon vanilla extract

2 tablespoons canola oil

½ cup water

Nonstick cooking spray

1. In a small saucepan over medium heat, mix the frozen berries and pomegranate juice together. Once the compote begins to boil, reduce the heat to low and simmer uncovered for 10 minutes, stirring occasionally.

2. In a large bowl, combine the buckwheat flour, self-rising flour, sugar, baking soda, cinnamon, and 1 teaspoon of chia seeds. Mix together.

3. In a medium bowl, whisk together the eggs, buttermilk, vanilla extract, oil, and water.

4. Make a well in the center of the dry ingredients and pour in the egg and buttermilk mixture. Stir until combined.

5. Spray a griddle or nonstick pan over medium-high heat with cooking spray. Pour ¼ cup of batter for each pancake. Cook for 2 to 3 minutes on one side, until small bubbles form in the batter, then flip and cook for an additional 1 to 2 minutes.

6. When the berry compote is ready, remove it from the heat and stir in the remaining 1 teaspoon of chia seeds. Allow to cool.

7. Serve pancakes topped with warm berry compote.

8. Store leftover pancakes for up to 3 days in the refrigerator and leftover compote for up to 1 week in the refrigerator.

SIMPLE SWAP: If you don't have self-rising flour, you can substitute ¾ cup all-purpose flour and 1½ teaspoons baking powder.

PER SERVING: Calories: 354; Total fat: 12g; Saturated fat: 2g; Sodium: 518mg; Carbohydrates: 52g; Fiber: 6g; Protein: 11g; Calcium: 202mg; Potassium: 359mg

BLUEBERRY-RICOTTA-STUFFED FRENCH TOAST

PREP TIME: 5 minutes   **COOK TIME:** 15 minutes

SERVES 4

Serve up a delicious brunch in the comfort of your home. Traditional stuffed French toast typically uses cream cheese or mascarpone cheese, both of which can be high in saturated fat. This lighter version uses protein-packed ricotta and flavoring from fresh blueberries to sweeten things up. Serve with additional fresh berries on the side for added fiber that will fuel you without overfilling you.

6 large eggs

¼ cup nonfat milk

¼ teaspoon vanilla extract

¼ teaspoon ground cinnamon

1 tablespoon butter or non-stick cooking spray

1 loaf brioche or challah bread, cut into 1-inch slices

1 cup part-skim ricotta cheese

1 cup fresh or defrosted frozen blueberries, divided

1. In a medium bowl, whisk together the eggs, milk, vanilla, and cinnamon. Set aside.

2. Preheat a griddle or nonstick pan over medium-high heat, and grease it with butter or cooking spray.

3. Dip the bread slices into the egg mixture to coat on both sides, then place on the griddle to cook for 3 to 5 minutes on each side, until browned.

4. Put the ricotta in a small bowl. Using a blender or food processor, puree ¼ cup of blueberries. Fold the blueberry puree into the ricotta cheese, then stir in the remaining ¾ cup of blueberries. Cover and refrigerate until ready to use.

5. Remove the bread from the griddle and spread ¼ cup of ricotta filling on one piece of bread, then top with another slice. Serve immediately.

6. Store leftover French toast in the refrigerator for up to 2 days or freeze for up to 3 months. The filling will keep for up to 2 or 3 days in the refrigerator. Store the filling and French toast separately, then reheat the bread and add the ricotta when serving.

SIMPLE SWAP: Swap the blueberries for any berry, such as strawberries or raspberries.

PER SERVING: Calories: 476; Total fat: 17g; Saturated fat: 8g; Sodium: 711mg; Carbohydrates: 53g; Fiber: 3g; Protein: 26g; Calcium: 280mg; Potassium: 330mg

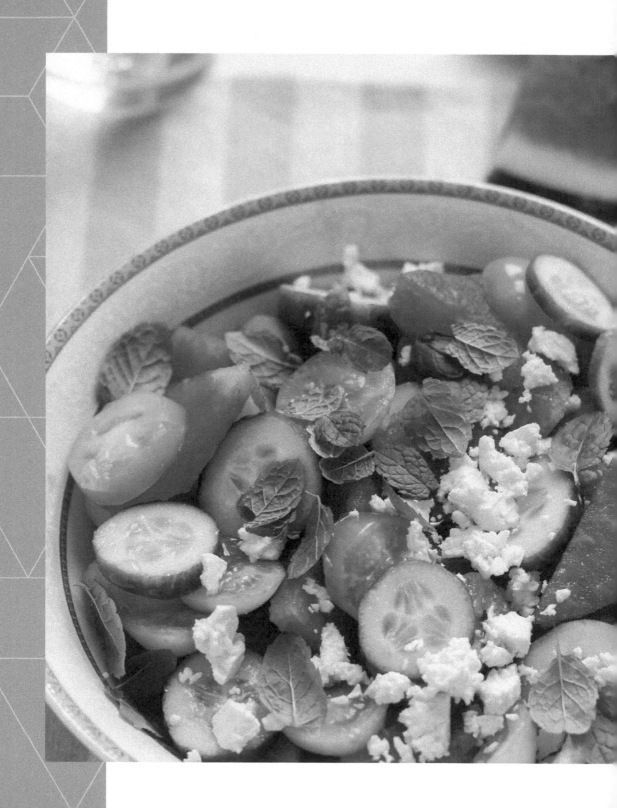

Salads and Bowls

Whenever someone tells me their typical lunchtime salad is lettuce with tomatoes, cucumbers, and grilled chicken, I cry a little inside. Salads can be fun, bright, colorful, inventive, and delicious. Healthy doesn't have to equal boring or bland. Bowls are also amazing. Basically, you can take any leftovers, arrange them in a bowl, and create a meal. Use the recipes in this chapter as a guideline for creating your own tasty bowls for appetizers, sides, or meals and, as a bonus, help reduce food waste.

KALE CAESAR SALAD

5-INGREDIENT   EXTRA LOW CALORIE
PREP TIME: 5 minutes   **COOK TIME:** 10 minutes
SERVES 2

This dairy-free Caesar salad slashes calories typically found in traditional versions. Nutritional yeast provides a cheesy flavor and adds protein, and a soft-boiled egg on top adds creaminess, thanks to the runny yolk. Raw kale can be tough, so giving it a massage with lemon juice and salt helps break down the fibers and make it more digestible.

2 large eggs

1 (10-ounce) bag washed, chopped kale

2 tablespoons extra-virgin olive oil

Juice of 1 lemon

¼ cup nutritional yeast, plus more for sprinkling if desired

2 tablespoons raw, shelled sunflower seeds

Kosher salt

Freshly ground black pepper

1. Bring a medium pot of water to a boil. Using a large slotted spoon, carefully lower the eggs into the water, separate from each other. Reduce the heat to a low simmer and boil for 6 to 8 minutes, depending on desired doneness of the yolk. Prepare an ice bath in a small bowl and set aside.

2. In a large bowl, combine the kale, olive oil, lemon juice, nutritional yeast, and sunflower seeds. Season with salt and pepper. Using your hands, massage the kale to combine it with the seasonings and soften the leaves.

3. Divide the kale greens between two plates. Top with additional nutritional yeast if desired.

4. Use the slotted spoon to transfer the eggs into the ice bath for 1 minute. Gently peel away the shells under cold running water, and top the kale greens with the soft-boiled eggs. Season with additional salt and pepper and enjoy immediately.

COOKING HACK: Wear latex gloves while massaging the kale for easier cleanup and reduced risk of cross-contamination.

PER SERVING: Calories: 347; Total fat: 24g; Saturated fat: 4g; Sodium: 216mg; Carbohydrates: 18g; Fiber: 7g; Protein: 18g; Calcium: 252mg; Potassium: 978mg

WATERMELON, TOMATO, CUCUMBER, FETA, AND MINT SALAD

EXTRA LOW CALORIE   ONE-POT

PREP TIME: 5 minutes

SERVES 4

Not every salad has to contain lettuce. This simple salad is one of my summer favorites. It's refreshing, and it involves seasonal warm-weather produce at its peak. I recommend using feta cheese that comes in a block, since it's more flavorful than crumbled feta. A premade balsamic glaze finishes the salad, providing a sweet complement to the salty feta cheese.

4 cups seedless watermelon, cubed

3 cups red or yellow grape tomatoes, halved

½ seedless English cucumber, sliced

1 (8-ounce) block feta cheese, diced

¼ cup fresh mint leaves, sliced

Balsamic glaze, for topping

Sea salt (optional)

Freshly ground black pepper (optional)

1. In a large bowl, toss the watermelon, tomatoes, cucumbers, feta cheese, and mint together.

2. Divide the mixture among four plates. Drizzle with balsamic glaze. Season with sea salt and pepper (if using).

SIMPLE SWAP: Fresh basil leaves can be used in place of the mint. When in season during the summer, try chopped heirloom or beefsteak tomatoes in place of the grape tomatoes.

PER SERVING: Calories: 225; Total fat: 13g; Saturated fat: 9g; Sodium: 529mg; Carbohydrates: 20g; Fiber: 2g; Protein: 10g; Calcium: 309mg; Potassium: 532mg

BEET, GOAT CHEESE, AND PISTACHIO SALAD

5-INGREDIENT   EXTRA LOW CALORIE   ONE-POT
PREP TIME: 5 minutes
SERVES 4

This simple and tasty salad pairs fiber- and antioxidant-rich beets with protein from goat cheese and pistachios. Precooked beets come to the rescue for this quick salad, which is perfect on its own or served as a side dish, such as with the Grilled Chicken Thighs Sandwich (page 101).

4 cups mixed greens

1 (6.5-ounce) package cooked beets, quartered

¼ cup crumbled goat cheese

2 tablespoons chopped shelled pistachios

½ cup Lemon-Shallot Champagne Vinaigrette (page 136) or any store-bought lemon vinaigrette

Divide the mixed greens among four plates. Top with the beets and goat cheese and sprinkle with the chopped pistachios. Drizzle with the vinaigrette.

COOKING HACK: Place the pistachios in a zip-top bag, squeeze out the air, and seal. Use a meat tenderizer or rolling pin to crush the pistachios.

PER SERVING: Calories: 138; Total fat: 10g; Saturated fat: 2g; Sodium: 363mg; Carbohydrates: 10g; Fiber: 2g; Protein: 4g; Calcium: 44mg; Potassium: 337mg

TANGY NO-MAYO TUNA SALAD

EXTRA LOW CALORIE   ONE-POT
PREP TIME: 10 minutes
SERVES 6

I was shocked when I first found out how many calories are in traditional deli tuna salad. This version puts a lighter Mediterranean spin on tuna salad by using vinegar, citrus juice, and heart-healthy olive oil instead of mayo. I've added crunchy veggies and Kalamata olives for a tangy twist loaded with antioxidants. This salad comes together in minutes with pantry and refrigerator staples—perfect for a quick lunch!

2 (12-ounce) cans albacore tuna in water, drained

½ cup chopped mini sweet bell peppers

¼ cup diced celery

2 tablespoons pitted, sliced Kalamata olives

2 tablespoons white wine vinegar

Juice of 1 lemon

1 tablespoon extra-virgin olive oil

½ teaspoon freshly ground black pepper

¼ teaspoon kosher salt

1. In a large bowl, combine the tuna, peppers, celery, olives, vinegar, lemon juice, olive oil, pepper, and salt. Use a fork to mix all the ingredients together.

2. Store leftover tuna salad in the refrigerator for up to 5 days.

SERVING SUGGESTION: Enjoy this tuna salad on its own, over mixed greens, as a sandwich or wrap, or with whole-grain crackers.

PER SERVING: Calories: 112; Total fat: 4g; Saturated fat: 1g; Sodium: 310mg; Carbohydrates: 2g; Fiber: 0g; Protein: 19g; Calcium: 22mg; Potassium: 217mg

WALDORF CHICKEN SALAD
LETTUCE WRAPS

EXTRA LOW CALORIE
PREP TIME: 20 minutes
SERVES 6

Possibilities abound for what you can do with store-cooked rotisserie chicken. My favorite use is chicken salad. This lightened-up version of the classic Waldorf salad uses Greek yogurt and olive oil mayo, which is lower in saturated fat than regular mayo. This is served on Bibb lettuce leaves for a low-carb wrap.

2 cups chopped
    cooked chicken

½ red apple (such as
    Honeycrisp), diced

½ cup red seedless
    grapes, halved

½ cup diced celery

½ cup chopped walnuts

½ cup plain nonfat
    Greek yogurt

¼ cup olive oil mayonnaise

1 teaspoon dried tarragon

⅛ teaspoon salt

⅛ teaspoon freshly ground
    black pepper

1 head Bibb lettuce

1. In a large bowl, combine the chicken, apples, grapes, celery, and walnuts.

2. In a small bowl, whisk together the yogurt, mayonnaise, tarragon, salt, and pepper. Add to the chicken salad mixture and stir to coat.

3. Serve the chicken salad with Bibb lettuce leaves to create wraps.

4. Store any leftover chicken salad in an airtight container in the refrigerator for up to 5 days.

SERVING SUGGESTION: Instead of lettuce wraps, enjoy a scoop of chicken salad over mixed greens or on whole-grain bread. You can also enjoy a simple snack of chicken salad on whole-grain crackers.

PER SERVING: Calories: 205; Total fat: 12g; Saturated fat: 2g; Sodium: 168mg; Carbohydrates: 8g; Fiber: 2g; Protein: 17g; Calcium: 53mg; Potassium: 315mg

GRILLED HALLOUMI SALAD

PREP TIME: 10 minutes   **COOK TIME:** 5 minutes
SERVES 4

I was recently introduced to Halloumi cheese and was fascinated to see that it can be placed directly on the grill and still maintain its shape. Halloumi makes a great vegetarian protein option, providing 7 grams of protein per ounce, and is an excellent source of calcium. The saltiness of the cheese complements the crunchy sweet fruits and nuts for a tasty mealtime salad.

Nonstick cooking spray

8 ounces Halloumi cheese, cut into ½-inch slices

2 cups mixed greens

½ red apple (such as Honeycrisp), thinly sliced

¼ cup pecan halves

¼ cup pomegranate arils

½ cup Lemon-Shallot Champagne Vinaigrette (page 136) or any store-bought vinaigrette

1. Preheat a grill pan or 10-inch nonstick skillet over medium-high heat. Spray with cooking spray. Place the Halloumi slices on the pan and cook for 3 minutes per side, until lightly browned and softened.

2. Divide the mixed greens among four bowls. Top with the apple slices, pecans, and pomegranate arils. Top with the grilled Halloumi and drizzle the vinaigrette on top.

COOKING HACK: Save time (and mess) by purchasing packages of fresh pomegranate arils in the refrigerated section of the produce department, or use frozen ones. Alternatively, swap with dried cherries or cranberries.

PER SERVING: Calories: 291; Total fat: 23g; Saturated fat: 10g; Sodium: 431mg; Carbohydrates: 13g; Fiber: 2g; Protein: 9g; Calcium: 300mg; Potassium: 204mg

ROASTED DELICATA SQUASH, CRANBERRY, AND GORGONZOLA SALAD

EXTRA LOW CALORIE   ONE-POT
PREP TIME: 5 minutes   **COOK TIME:** 20 minutes
SERVES 4

This colorful salad exemplifies fall in a bowl. Delicata squashes are easier to cut than most hard-skinned winter squashes, and they cook quickly. Roasting brings out their natural sweetness. I've combined the squash with peppery arugula, sweet cranberries, crunchy protein-rich pepitas, and tangy Gorgonzola cheese. For a milder cheese, swap in goat or feta cheese.

1 large delicata squash

1 tablespoon olive oil

1 tablespoon honey

½ teaspoon dried thyme

Salt

Freshly ground black pepper

4 cups arugula

¼ cup dried cranberries

¼ cup unsalted pepitas

¼ cup Gorgonzola cheese

½ cup Raspberry–Poppy Seed Dressing (page 137)

1. Preheat the oven to 425°F and line a sheet pan with nonstick aluminum foil.

2. Slice off the ends of the squash, then cut the squash in half lengthwise. Use a spoon to scoop out the seeds. Place the halves flat-sides down and cut into ¼-inch slices.

3. In a zip-top bag, combine the squash with the olive oil, honey, and thyme and shake to coat. Remove the squash from the bag, spread it in a single layer on the sheet pan, season with salt and pepper, and roast for 20 minutes, turning halfway through.

4. Divide the arugula among four bowls and top with the dried cranberries, pepitas, and Gorgonzola. Add the roasted squash and drizzle with the dressing.

5. Store leftover salad without dressing in the refrigerator for up to 2 days.

LOVE YOUR LEFTOVERS: Save the delicata seeds to roast for a tasty snack! Toss the seeds with olive oil and seasonings. Roast at 375°F for 8 to 10 minutes, tossing every few minutes to prevent burning.

PER SERVING: Calories: 220; Total fat: 12g; Saturated fat: 3g; Sodium: 431mg; Carbohydrates: 27g; Fiber: 3g; Protein: 5g; Calcium: 122mg; Potassium: 561mg

COLD SESAME NOODLE BOWL

5-INGREDIENT   **EXTRA LOW CALORIE**
PREP TIME: 5 minutes   **COOK TIME:** 5 minutes
SERVES 4

Noodle bowls are a popular take-out item, but they're so easy to make at home. This version saves on both calories and sodium content and boosts the protein with plant protein from edamame. Frozen edamame is a fantastic freezer staple to keep handy for a quick source of protein. If you'd like, top your bowl with additional protein or vegetables such as thinly sliced bell peppers, cucumber, or shredded red cabbage.

1 (10-ounce package) udon or soba noodles

½ cup Sesame, Miso, and Ginger Dressing (page 139) or store-bought dressing

1 cup frozen shelled edamame, thawed

¼ cup scallions, thinly sliced

2 tablespoons sesame seeds, toasted (see Technique Trick)

1. Bring a pot of water to a boil and cook the noodles according to the package directions. Drain and rinse under cold water.

2. Return the noodles to the pot. Add the dressing and stir until coated. Add the edamame, scallions, and sesame seeds and toss together to mix the noodles and dressing. Add additional dressing as needed. Divide into bowls, add any desired additional toppings, and serve.

3. Store leftover noodles in the refrigerator for up to 5 days.

TECHNIQUE TRICK: To toast the sesame seeds, place them in a small ungreased nonstick skillet over medium-high heat. Gently shake the pan frequently to toss the seeds and prevent sticking or burning. Cook until they turn brown and fragrant and begin to release oils, 2 to 3 minutes.

PER SERVING: Calories: 383; Total fat: 11g; Saturated fat: 2g; Sodium: 631mg; Carbohydrates: 61g; Fiber: 3g; Protein: 15g; Calcium: 60mg; Potassium: 404mg

CAULIFLOWER RICE BURRITO BOWL

PREP TIME: 5 minutes   **COOK TIME:** 10 minutes
SERVES 2

I've often encouraged clients to choose burrito bowls or salads if they enjoy Tex-Mex takeout, to help save on calories and carbs and load up on veggies. This deconstructed burrito in a bowl enlists high-fiber cauliflower rice topped with veggies and beans to provide plant-based protein. Optionally, you can top your bowl with avocado, jalapeños, mango, or any additional protein to customize your bowl.

1 (15.5-ounce) can black beans, drained and rinsed

1 cup frozen corn

1 (14.5-ounce) can diced tomatoes, drained with juices reserved

½ teaspoon chili powder

½ teaspoon cumin

1 tablespoon avocado oil

1 (12-ounce) bag cauliflower rice

¼ teaspoon kosher salt

¼ cup chopped cilantro, plus more for sprinkling if desired

Juice of 1 lime

¼ cup shredded cheddar Jack cheese

1. In a small saucepan over medium heat, combine the beans, frozen corn, tomatoes, 2 tablespoons of the reserved tomato juice, chili powder, and cumin. Cook for 3 to 5 minutes, stirring occasionally, until heated through.

2. In a large nonstick skillet over medium heat, heat the avocado oil. Add the cauliflower rice and salt. Sauté for 3 to 5 minutes, stirring occasionally, until heated through and slightly tender. Remove from the heat and stir in the cilantro and lime juice.

3. Divide the cauliflower rice between two bowls and top with the bean mixture and shredded cheese. Sprinkle with chopped cilantro or other toppings, if desired.

LOVE YOUR LEFTOVERS: Scramble eggs with any remaining bean, corn, and tomato mixture for a quick breakfast, or use it as filling for Chicken and Black Bean Quesadillas (page 102).

PER SERVING: Calories: 461; Total fat: 14g; Saturated fat: 4g; Sodium: 558mg; Carbohydrates: 71g; Fiber: 22g; Protein: 23g; Calcium: 302mg; Potassium: 1,815mg

PESTO GRAIN BOWL WITH CHICKPEAS

PREP TIME: 5 minutes   **COOK TIME:** 15 minutes

SERVES 4

Grain bowls are a fancy way to use up leftovers. I always keep cooked grains on hand for quick side dishes. When lunchtime comes around, I simply combine my grains with any veggies I have available. This colorful bowl includes chickpeas, a pantry staple and an easy way to add protein. In addition to quinoa, you may also want to try this recipe with other grains, such as sorghum or farro.

1 cup uncooked quinoa

1½ cups chicken or vegetable broth

1 large zucchini, diced

1 cup grape tomatoes, halved

1 (15.5-ounce) can chickpeas, drained and rinsed

1 (8-ounce) container small pearl-size mozzarella balls, drained

¼ cup Spinach-Pistachio Pesto Sauce (page 140) or any store-bought pesto sauce, plus 2 tablespoons

1. Cook the quinoa in the broth according to package directions.

2. In a large bowl, combine the zucchini, tomatoes, chickpeas, and mozzarella balls. Stir in ¼ cup of pesto sauce to coat.

3. After the quinoa is cooked, stir in the remaining 2 tablespoons of pesto sauce.

4. Divide the quinoa among four bowls and top with the vegetable, chickpea, and mozzarella mixture.

5. Store any leftover grain bowl in the refrigerator for up to 3 days.

COOKING HACK: Look for precooked quinoa in the rice or grains section of the grocery store. These packages can be microwaved in 90 seconds, cutting down on cooking time.

PER SERVING: Calories: 560; Total fat: 30g; Saturated fat: 10g; Sodium: 741mg; Carbohydrates: 47g; Fiber: 8g; Protein: 27g; Calcium: 408mg; Potassium: 703mg

FALAFEL BOWL

EXTRA LOW CALORIE

PREP TIME: 10 minutes   **COOK TIME:** 15 minutes
SERVES 6

Falafel are traditionally deep-fried chickpea balls served in pita. Air-frying the falafel makes this a healthy protein topping to a traditional Greek salad. No air fryer? No problem! Just bake the falafel instead (see Cooking Hack). You can also top this bowl with chopped tomatoes, cucumbers, Kalamata olives, and feta cheese.

2 (15.5-ounce) cans chickpeas, drained and rinsed

2 garlic cloves

¼ cup fresh parsley

¼ cup fresh cilantro

1 teaspoon cumin

½ teaspoon salt

½ teaspoon freshly ground black pepper

¼ cup panko bread crumbs

1 to 2 tablespoons water

Nonstick cooking spray

6 cups chopped romaine lettuce

¾ cup Tzatziki Sauce (page 141) or store-bought tzatziki sauce

1. In a food processor, combine the chickpeas, garlic, parsley, cilantro, cumin, salt, and pepper. Pulse a few times to combine, scraping down the sides. Add the panko and pulse again to combine. Add the water if the mixture is too dry and crumbly.

2. Make 2-tablespoon-size balls using your hands. Place the falafel in the air fryer basket, spray with cooking spray, and cook for 15 minutes at 400°F until browned, flipping halfway.

3. Divide the romaine among six bowls. Top each bowl with three falafels and any additional toppings if desired, and drizzle tzatziki sauce on top.

4. Store leftover falafel in the refrigerator for up to 5 days. Store the romaine without dressing in the refrigerator for up to 3 days.

COOKING HACK: If you don't have an air fryer, bake the falafel on a sheet pan lined with parchment paper in a 425°F oven for 15 to 20 minutes.

PER SERVING: Calories: 127; Total fat: 3g; Saturated fat: 0g; Sodium: 366mg; Carbohydrates: 20g; Fiber: 6g; Protein: 7g; Calcium: 72mg; Potassium: 265mg

SUNFLOWER TACO SALAD BOWL

ONE-POT
PREP TIME: 15 minutes
SERVES 4

A local vegan restaurant opened my eyes to using sunflower seeds as taco meat. An amazing source of protein, sunflower seeds provide almost 30 grams of protein per cup, along with healthy fats and antioxidants. This vegetarian taco salad comes together in minutes and will surprise any meat eater.

1 cup raw, shelled sunflower seeds

2 tablespoons taco seasoning

4 cups chopped romaine lettuce

1 cup shredded red cabbage

1 avocado, peeled, pitted, and diced

1 cup diced Oaxaca cheese or shredded four-cheese Mexican blend

½ cup fresh refrigerated salsa or pico de gallo

½ cup Avocado Buttermilk Ranch Dressing (page 138) or store-bought Greek yogurt–based ranch dressing (such as Bolthouse Farms)

1. In a small bowl of water, soak the sunflower seeds for 10 minutes. Drain the seeds and place in a food processor or blender with the taco seasoning. Pulse until combined and the texture is crumbly and resembles ground meat.

2. Divide the romaine lettuce among four bowls. Top with the shredded cabbage, sunflower taco meat, avocado, cheese, salsa, and ranch dressing.

3. Store any leftover sunflower taco meat in the refrigerator for up to 5 days.

SIMPLE SWAP: Instead of a bowl, create low-carb tacos by using collard leaves in place of tortillas.

PER SERVING: Calories: 429; Total fat: 32g; Saturated fat: 7g; Sodium: 632mg; Carbohydrates: 24g; Fiber: 9g; Protein: 15g; Calcium: 256mg; Potassium: 770mg

CRISPY TOFU BOWL

PREP TIME: 10 minutes   **COOK TIME:** 15 minutes
SERVES 4

An amazing source of plant-based protein, tofu takes on the flavor of whatever you cook it in. Crispy tofu is a good introduction to tofu if you're not used to eating it. This recipe uses an air fryer to crisp the tofu, but you can also bake or sauté it (see Cooking Hack). For even more crunch, garnish these bowls with sliced almonds or sesame seeds.

1 cup uncooked jasmine rice

1 (14-ounce) block extra-firm tofu, drained

2 tablespoons low-sodium soy sauce

1 tablespoon white miso

1 tablespoon sesame oil

Nonstick cooking spray

1 cup shredded carrots

1 cup thinly sliced mini sweet bell peppers

1 cup shredded red cabbage

¼ cup sliced scallions

½ cup Sesame, Miso, and Ginger Dressing (page 139)

1. Cook the rice according to the package directions and set aside.

2. Wrap the tofu in layers of paper towels and press to release the excess liquid. Place a heavy-bottomed pot on top to continue pressing out the liquid.

3. In a large bowl, whisk together the soy sauce, miso, and sesame oil until smooth.

4. Cut the tofu into 1-inch cubes, add them to the large bowl, and toss to coat with the sauce.

5. Layer the tofu in the air fryer basket, spray with cooking spray, and cook for 15 minutes at 400°F, tossing halfway through.

6. Divide the rice among four bowls and top with the carrots, bell peppers, cabbage, and scallions. Add the tofu and drizzle with the dressing.

7. Store leftover bowls in the refrigerator for up to 1 day.

COOKING HACK: If you don't have an air fryer, bake the tofu on a sheet pan lined with parchment paper in a 425°F oven for 15 to 20 minutes or sauté in a large nonstick pan coated with 1 tablespoon oil until browned on all sides.

PER SERVING: Calories: 404; Total fat: 16g; Saturated fat: 2g; Sodium: 541mg; Carbohydrates: 51g; Fiber: 3g; Protein: 15g; Calcium: 240mg; Potassium: 478mg

SALMON TERIYAKI POWER BOWL

PREP TIME: 5 minutes   **COOK TIME:** 10 minutes
SERVES 4

Create a restaurant-quality power bowl from the comfort of your home. Short-cuts like precooked rice, prepared veggies, frozen edamame, and store-bought low-sodium teriyaki sauce (I recommend Kikkoman) bring this meal together in record time.

2 (8-ounce) packages precooked brown rice

4 (4-ounce) skinless salmon fillets

¾ cup teriyaki sauce, divided, plus more for drizzling

1 pound sliced shiitake or cremini mushrooms

1 cup frozen shelled edamame, thawed

1 cup shredded red cabbage

⅔ cup shredded carrots

2 tablespoons sliced scallions (optional)

1. Preheat the oven broiler on high and line a sheet pan with nonstick aluminum foil.

2. Microwave the brown rice according to the package instructions and set aside.

3. In a large bowl or zip-top bag, toss the salmon with ½ cup of teriyaki sauce.

4. In a separate small bowl or bag, toss the mushrooms with the remaining ¼ cup of teriyaki sauce.

5. Place the salmon on the lined sheet pan and reserve the remaining sauce. Broil the salmon for 3 minutes. Remove from the broiler, flip the salmon, brush on the reserved teriyaki sauce, scatter the mushrooms around the salmon, and broil for an additional 2 minutes.

6. Among four bowls, divide the rice, edamame, cabbage, and carrots. Top with the broiled salmon and mushrooms. Sprinkle the scallions on top (if using). Drizzle with additional teriyaki sauce if desired.

7. Store leftover salmon separately from the rice and vegetables. Reheat the salmon in the oven or broiler for 3 to 5 minutes. Enjoy the rice and vegetables cold or microwave for 1 to 2 minutes to warm.

SIMPLE SWAP: Frozen salmon can be used in place of fresh. If the fillets come with skin, start by broiling the fillets skin-side up. Shrimp or tuna can be swapped for the salmon; alternatively, use tofu for a vegetarian version.

PER SERVING: Calories: 441; Total fat: 10g; Saturated fat: 2g; Sodium: 716mg; Carbohydrates: 50g; Fiber: 8g; Protein: 38g; Calcium: 108mg; Potassium: 1,317mg

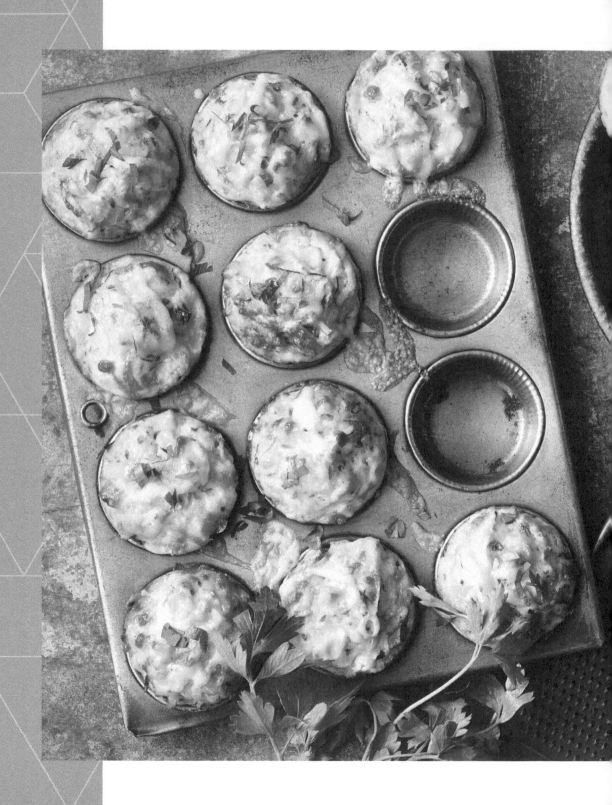

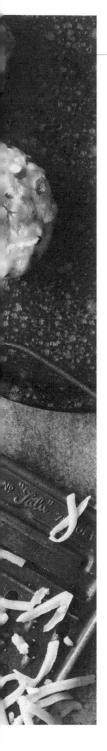

CHAPTER FOUR

Breads, Muffins, and Yummy Carbs

You may be wondering how a chapter dedicated to carbs wound up in a weight-loss book. Here's the thing: Carbs are our main source of fuel. Carbs aren't bad for us, they're just misunderstood. It all comes down to quality and quantity of foods, and carbs are no exception. From side dishes to main meals, carbs can be enjoyed in a range of dishes that shouldn't be feared but embraced. Enjoy these carbs while keeping portion sizes in check, and pair them with lean proteins. If you choose to enjoy a yummy carb on its own, savor it.

GREEK YOGURT BAGEL BITES

5-INGREDIENT   EXTRA LOW CALORIE
PREP TIME: 15 minutes   **COOK TIME:** 15 minutes
SERVES 6

As a Jersey girl, I consider myself a bagel connoisseur. When I discovered a way to create fluffy bagels at home in under 30 minutes, even my husband—a fellow bagel snob—was impressed. These bagel bites provide a small bagel fix and are a perfect complement to egg dishes, such as the Sheet Pan Veggie Hash (page 30). Or enjoy with a spread of Pea Hummus (page 146), whipped cream cheese, Neufchâtel cheese, or smashed avocado on top, along with some slices of lox, cucumber, or tomato.

Nonstick cooking spray

2 cups self-rising flour, plus more for dusting

1½ cups plain nonfat Greek yogurt

1 large egg, separated, or 3 tablespoons liquid egg whites

1 tablespoon water

Everything bagel seasoning blend, for topping (optional)

1. Preheat the oven to 400°F. Line a sheet pan with parchment paper and spray with cooking spray.

2. In a large bowl, combine the flour, yogurt, and egg yolk (if using) until a soft dough forms. Use your hands to form the dough into a large ball.

3. Turn the dough out onto a floured surface and knead it, generously adding flour as needed to prevent sticking. The dough should be smooth and elastic and will require 8 to 10 kneading turns.

4. Using a rounded tablespoon scoop, create dough balls about the size of a golf ball and place them on the prepared sheet pan, at least 1 inch apart.

5. Whisk together the egg white with the water. Brush the egg wash on top and sprinkle with everything bagel seasoning blend (if using).

6. Place the pan on the top oven rack and bake for 15 to 18 minutes, until the tops are browned. Let cool before enjoying.

7. Store bagels in a plastic zip-top bag at room temperature for up to 5 days or freeze for up to 3 months.

COOKING HACK: Cut down on kneading time by using an electric mixer with a dough hook attachment.

PER SERVING: Calories: 197; Total fat: 2g; Saturated fat: 0g; Sodium: 530mg; Carbohydrates: 33g; Fiber: 1g; Protein: 11g; Calcium: 208mg; Potassium: 143mg

IRISH SODA BREAD SCONES

PREP TIME: 10 minutes   **COOK TIME:** 20 minutes
SERVES 12

When I was growing up, I always knew it was the holidays when I could smell my mom baking her Irish soda bread. This recipe is still a fan favorite in my household. The original recipe creates a large loaf and takes over an hour to bake. Creating smaller scone versions bakes them faster and makes smaller portions that you can freeze as leftovers for another time.

5 cups all-purpose flour, divided, plus more for dusting

1 cup sugar

1 teaspoon baking soda

1 teaspoon salt

1⅓ cups buttermilk

1 cup raisins

12 tablespoons (1½ sticks) unsalted butter, melted

1. Preheat the oven to 425°F. Line a sheet pan with parchment paper. Place 1 cup of flour in a small bowl and set aside.

2. In a large bowl, stir together the remaining 4 cups of flour, sugar, baking soda, and salt. Form a well in the center and add the buttermilk, raisins, and butter. Stir together to form a dough. The dough will be slightly crumbly.

3. Turn the dough out onto a floured surface and knead the bread until smooth and no longer sticky. Flatten the kneaded dough to create a rectangle. Create scoops of dough using a ⅓ measuring cup. Place the measuring cup upside down on the dough so the opening is toward the dough. Press down to cut into the dough and create a rounded biscuit-like shape.

4. Lightly roll each scone in the remaining flour and place on the prepared sheet pan, 2 inches apart.

5. Bake for 20 minutes. Remove from the oven and allow to cool before enjoying.

6. Store leftover scones in a plastic zip-top bag at room temperature for up to 2 days, in the refrigerator for up 1 week, or in the freezer for up to 3 months.

SERVING SUGGESTION: These scones can be enjoyed on their own with jam or Irish butter. Serve with eggs and fruit for added protein and fiber.

PER SERVING: Calories: 403; Total fat: 13g; Saturated fat: 8g; Sodium: 355mg; Carbohydrates: 68g; Fiber: 2g; Protein: 7g; Calcium: 49mg; Potassium: 191mg

CHEESY GARLIC PULL-APART BREADSTICKS

EXTRA LOW CALORIE   ONE-POT
PREP TIME: 10 minutes   **COOK TIME:** 10 minutes
SERVES 4

When I was in college, there was a pizza shop that made a very unhealthy version of these breadsticks, which I believe was a major contributor to the "Freshman 15" weight gain. They were made with so much butter and oil, you could practically see through the box. These yummy breadsticks contain a lot less oil, no butter, and low-fat cheese. Enjoy along with a lean protein and salad for balance.

Nonstick cooking spray

1 teaspoon grated Parmesan cheese

4 garlic cloves, minced

½ teaspoon dried parsley, plus more for topping if desired

½ teaspoon dried oregano, plus more for topping if desired

¼ teaspoon onion powder

¼ cup olive oil

1 premade pizza dough

¾ cup shredded part-skim mozzarella cheese

1. Preheat the oven to 450°F. Line a sheet pan with parchment paper and spray with cooking spray.

2. In a small bowl, combine the Parmesan cheese, garlic, parsley, oregano, and onion powder. Mix together. Add the olive oil and stir to combine.

3. Shape the pizza dough on the sheet pan to a 12- to 14-inch diameter round crust. Using a pastry brush or the back of a spoon, brush the garlic-oil mixture on the crust in a thin layer. Top with the shredded mozzarella cheese. Sprinkle on additional parsley and oregano, if desired.

4. Bake on the lowest oven rack for 10 to 12 minutes, until the edges are browned and the cheese is bubbling.

5. Remove from the oven. Using a pizza cutter or knife, cut the crust in half lengthwise, then cut across in the other direction, creating 1½-inch-wide sticks.

SERVING SUGGESTION: These sticks are designed to be dipped, so serve along with your favorite dipping sauce, such as marinara.

PER SERVING: Calories: 319; Total fat: 19g; Saturated fat: 4g; Sodium: 498mg; Carbohydrates: 28g; Fiber: 2g; Protein: 10g; Calcium: 190mg; Potassium: 35mg

JALAPEÑO-CHEDDAR CORN MUFFINS

EXTRA LOW CALORIE

PREP TIME: 10 minutes   **COOK TIME:** 15 minutes
SERVES 6

Corn muffins are one of my favorite savory muffins, and when you add cheese and a little spice, it's a bonus. These easily prepared muffins make a tasty complement to meals. Get a batch going to serve along with Turkey Chili (page 87) or Chicken Chorizo and Egg Breakfast Skillet (page 33) or just to enjoy on their own.

Nonstick cooking spray (optional)

2 jalapeños

1 cup all-purpose flour

1 cup yellow cornmeal

2 tablespoons sugar

1 tablespoon baking powder

½ teaspoon salt

2 large eggs, lightly beaten

1 cup nonfat milk

4 tablespoons (½ stick) unsalted butter, melted

2 tablespoons honey

1 cup shredded cheddar cheese

1. Preheat the oven to 375°F. Line a 12-cup muffin tin with paper liners or coat with cooking spray.

2. Cut one jalapeño pepper in half lengthwise to remove the seeds and ribs. Chop the pepper into thin half-moon shapes. Set aside. Slice the other jalapeño into thin rounds and set aside separately.

3. In a large bowl, mix together the flour, cornmeal, sugar, baking powder, salt, eggs, milk, butter, and honey until combined. Add the half-moon jalapeño slices and cheese, stirring until the batter is well blended.

4. Pour ¼ cup of batter into each muffin cup. Top each with round jalapeño slices. Bake for 12 to 15 minutes, until the tops are browned and domed and a toothpick inserted into the center of a muffin comes out clean. Allow to cool completely before enjoying.

5. Store in an airtight container at room temperature for 2 days, in the refrigerator for up to 1 week, or in the freezer for up to 2 months.

COOKING HACK: Use a boxed corn muffin mix to cut down on prep time. Add the honey, jalapeños, and cheddar to the mix and bake according to package instructions.

PER SERVING: Calories: 374; Total fat: 17g; Saturated fat: 9g; Sodium: 372mg; Carbohydrates: 45g; Fiber: 2g; Protein: 12g; Calcium: 305mg; Potassium: 458mg

MINI PUMPKIN–CHOCOLATE CHIP MUFFINS

EXTRA LOW CALORIE

PREP TIME: 15 minutes   **COOK TIME:** 15 minutes
SERVES 12

When it comes to yummy carbs, these are it. The mini size helps with portion control and satisfies a sweet tooth. I consider these a great mindfulness treat, as you can get a lot of pleasure from even just a small bite. This recipe makes 36 mini muffins, so freeze extras to savor again later.

Nonstick cooking spray
  (optional)

1⅔ cups all-purpose flour

1 cup sugar

1 teaspoon pumpkin pie spice

1 teaspoon baking soda

¼ teaspoon baking powder

¼ teaspoon salt

2 large eggs

1 cup pumpkin puree

8 tablespoons (1 stick)
  unsalted butter, melted

1 cup mini chocolate chips

1. Preheat the oven to 375°F. Line two mini muffin pans with liners or grease with cooking spray.

2. In a large bowl, combine the flour, sugar, pumpkin pie spice, baking soda, baking powder, and salt.

3. In a medium bowl, whisk together the eggs, pumpkin puree, and melted butter.

4. Make a well in the center of the dry ingredients and pour in the wet ingredients. Add the chocolate chips. Stir to combine until mixed together.

5. Scoop 1 rounded tablespoon of batter into each mini muffin cup.

6. Place both muffin tins on the middle oven rack. If both muffin tins don't fit on the middle rack, switch the tins on the racks halfway through for even baking. Bake for 12 to 15 minutes, until browned and domed on top and a toothpick inserted in the center of a muffin comes out clean. Allow to cool before enjoying.

7. Store leftover muffins in a plastic zip-top bag at room temperature for up to 4 days or freeze for up to 3 months.

TECHNIQUE TRICK: If there is not enough batter to fill a full muffin tin at the end, fill the middle rows of the tin with the remaining mixture. Fill any empty muffin cups about a quarter full of water. This will help the muffins bake evenly.

PER SERVING (4 MINI MUFFINS): Calories: 251; Total fat: 11g; Saturated fat: 7g; Sodium: 169mg; Carbohydrates: 35g; Fiber: 2g; Protein: 4g; Calcium: 25mg; Potassium: 122mg

FIG, BLUE CHEESE, AND ARUGULA FLATBREAD

EXTRA LOW CALORIE   ONE-POT
PREP TIME: 5 minutes   **COOK TIME:** 10 minutes
SERVES 2 TO 4

I often refer to flatbreads as pizzas with more fun toppings. This combo of figs, blue cheese, and arugula is a perfect example. Make this flatbread for a quick sweet and savory lunch for two or as an appetizer for four. Using naan cuts down on time making your own crust, and whole-wheat options boost the fiber. However, any premade flatbread crust can be used if naan is unavailable.

2 pieces whole-wheat naan bread

¼ cup thinly sliced shallot

½ cup blue cheese crumbles

½ cup dried or fresh figs, quartered

1 tablespoon extra-virgin olive oil

1 teaspoon honey

Salt

Freshly ground black pepper

1 cup fresh arugula

Balsamic glaze, for topping

1. Preheat the oven to 400°F. Line a sheet pan with parchment paper.

2. Place the naan on the prepared sheet pan. Top the flatbread with shallots, blue cheese, and figs. Bake for 10 minutes, until the edges are brown and the cheese is melted.

3. In a small bowl, whisk together the olive oil and honey and season with salt and pepper to taste. Toss the arugula in the dressing to coat.

4. Remove the flatbread from the oven and top with the dressed arugula. Drizzle the balsamic glaze on top and serve immediately.

COOKING HACK: If you prefer a crispier crust, use a pizza stone or pizza crisper pan and bake on the bottom rack of the oven.

PER SERVING (AS A MEAL): Calories: 151; Total fat: 6g; Saturated fat: 3g; Sodium: 242mg; Carbohydrates: 20g; Fiber: 2g; Protein: 5g; Calcium: 81mg; Potassium: 160mg

BUTTERNUT SQUASH
MAC AND CHEESE

ONE-POT

PREP TIME: 10 minutes   **COOK TIME:** 20 minutes
SERVES 4

Nothing says comfort food more than mac and cheese, but mac and cheese can also be a high-calorie ticket item, especially if it comes from a box. This lightened-up version gets its creaminess and flavor from butternut squash, which also boosts the nutritional value for a healthier comfort food option. It all comes together in one pot for a no-fuss meal.

1 (16-ounce) bag frozen butternut squash

1 tablespoon olive oil

3 garlic cloves, minced

2 cups low-sodium chicken broth

1 cup nonfat milk

½ teaspoon dried thyme

¼ teaspoon salt

¼ teaspoon freshly ground black pepper

8 ounces small shell pasta (2 cups dry)

1 cup shredded cheddar cheese

1. Thaw the butternut squash in the microwave by cooking according to package directions. Once thawed, create a puree using a potato masher or fork.

2. In a medium pot, heat the oil over medium heat. Add the garlic and sauté for 30 seconds, until fragrant.

3. Add the butternut squash puree, broth, milk, thyme, salt, and pepper. Whisk to combine, increase the heat to medium-high, and bring to a boil, 5 minutes.

4. Once the sauce is bubbling, stir in the pasta. Cover, reduce heat to low, and simmer for 10 minutes, until the pasta is tender.

5. Remove the pot from the heat and stir in the cheese. Allow to cool for 5 minutes as the sauce thickens. The sauce will continue to thicken as it cools.

6. Store leftovers in the refrigerator for 3 to 5 days.

SIMPLE SWAP: Canned butternut squash, pumpkin puree, or frozen sweet potato can be swapped for the frozen butternut squash.

PER SERVING: Calories: 465; Total fat: 15g; Saturated fat: 6g; Sodium: 402mg; Carbohydrates: 64g; Fiber: 3g; Protein: 21g; Calcium: 324mg; Potassium: 606mg

TURKEY TACO–STUFFED SWEET POTATOES

EXTRA LOW CALORIE   ONE-POT
PREP TIME: 10 minutes   **COOK TIME:** 20 minutes
SERVES 4

Give your tacos a new vehicle by trading tortillas for sweet potatoes. You'll get a boost of nutrients from the sweet potato, including beta-carotene, vitamin C, and fiber. Top these with cheese, avocado, salsa, or any of your favorite taco toppings.

4 small sweet potatoes

1 tablespoon olive oil

1 cup diced sweet onion

½ yellow bell pepper, diced

1 pound ground turkey

2 tablespoons low-sodium taco seasoning

1 (14.5-ounce) can diced tomatoes, drained with juices reserved

1. Pierce the sweet potatoes several times with a fork. Place on a microwave-safe plate and microwave for 10 minutes, rotating halfway through, until the potatoes are tender.

2. Meanwhile, in a large nonstick skillet, heat the oil over medium-high heat. Add the onions and peppers and sauté, stirring occasionally, until the onions are translucent and the peppers are tender, 5 minutes.

3. Add the ground turkey and taco seasoning to the skillet and continue to sauté, breaking up the turkey meat and combining all the ingredients. Stir in ¼ cup of reserved tomato juice until absorbed. Continue to cook until the turkey meat is browned and no longer pink inside, 7 minutes.

4. Add the diced tomatoes and mix until combined. Add the remaining tomato juice and stir until absorbed. Remove from the heat.

5. Split the baked sweet potatoes down the middle lengthwise and then across to create a cross shape. Gently press the ends to puff out the sweet potatoes, and scoop out 2 tablespoons of the flesh to create a bowl. Fill with the turkey meat and top with toppings of your choice.

LOVE YOUR LEFTOVERS: Save the sweet potato flesh from the potatoes. This can be added into smoothies, stirred into oatmeal, or used to make a quick mashed sweet potato side dish.

PER SERVING: Calories: 327; Total fat: 12g; Saturated fat: 3g; Sodium: 395mg; Carbohydrates: 30g; Fiber: 6g; Protein: 25g; Calcium: 97mg; Potassium: 923mg

AIR-FRYER GNOCCHI WITH POMODORO SAUCE

5-INGREDIENT   EXTRA LOW CALORIE
PREP TIME: 5 minutes   **COOK TIME:** 20 minutes
SERVES 4

Air-frying gnocchi can turn anyone into a fan. My husband hated gnocchi until he tried it air-fried. The outside crisps up while the inside stays soft and fluffy. (See Cooking Hack for oven-cooking instructions.) This gnocchi gets paired with pomodoro sauce, which is a light tomato sauce with basil. This recipe works best with frozen cauliflower gnocchi or refrigerated potato gnocchi.

1 (28-ounce) can whole peeled tomatoes (Roma or San Marzano)

2 tablespoons olive oil

2 garlic cloves, minced

2 (10-ounce) bags frozen cauliflower gnocchi, or 16 ounces refrigerated potato gnocchi

Nonstick cooking spray

6 or 7 fresh basil leaves, sliced in thin strips

Ricotta or Parmesan cheese, for garnish (optional)

1. Empty the canned tomatoes into a large bowl and gently squeeze them with your hands to release their juices and create tomato chunks. Use a blender to puree the tomatoes if you prefer a thinner sauce.

2. In a medium pot, heat the olive oil over medium heat. Add the garlic and sauté for 30 seconds until fragrant. Add the tomatoes to the pot and stir together with the oil and garlic. Bring to a boil, then cover, reduce the heat to low, and allow the sauce to simmer for at least 20 minutes.

3. While the sauce simmers, place the gnocchi in a single layer in the air fryer basket. Spray with cooking spray and cook at 400°F for 10 to 12 minutes, tossing halfway through. The gnocchi will be browned and crisp when done.

4. Stir the basil into the sauce just before serving. Serve the gnocchi topped with the pomodoro sauce. If desired, garnish the gnocchi with a dollop of ricotta cheese or a sprinkle of Parmesan cheese.

COOKING HACK: If you don't own an air fryer, the gnocchi can be cooked in the oven. Toss the gnocchi in 1 tablespoon olive oil and place on a sheet pan lined with parchment paper or a baking rack. Bake at 425°F for 20 minutes, or until browned and crisp, stirring halfway through.

PER SERVING: Calories: 132; Total fat: 8g; Saturated fat: 1g; Sodium: 63mg; Carbohydrates: 15g; Fiber: 7g; Protein: 4g; Calcium: 101mg; Potassium: 811mg

RAVIOLI AND SPINACH BAKED SKILLET

5-INGREDIENT   EXTRA LOW CALORIE   ONE-POT
PREP TIME: 5 minutes   **COOK TIME:** 15 minutes
SERVES 4

I used to avoid making pasta dishes because it dirtied so many pots and pans. This skillet meal changes that—everything cooks in one pan. Refrigerated ravioli cooks in minutes right in the store-bought marinara (I recommend Rao's). This recipe calls for mozzarella cheese ravioli, but it can work with any cheese or veggie-filled variety.

1 (24-ounce) jar marinara sauce

2 cups fresh baby spinach

1 (20-ounce) package refrigerated small mozzarella cheese ravioli

1 cup shredded part-skim mozzarella cheese

1 tablespoon chopped fresh basil

1. Preheat the oven to 375°F.

2. Heat a large, oven-safe nonstick skillet over medium-high heat. Combine the marinara and spinach in the skillet. Bring to a boil and stir until the spinach is wilted, 3 to 5 minutes.

3. Add the ravioli and stir until coated. Allow to cook for 2 to 3 minutes, until heated through, stirring occasionally to prevent sticking. Spread the ravioli into a single layer in the skillet and spread the cheese on top. Place in the oven and bake for 5 minutes, until the cheese is melted and bubbling. Carefully remove from the oven. Top with fresh basil and serve.

4. Store leftover baked ravioli in the refrigerator for 3 to 5 days.

SIMPLE SWAP: Frozen ravioli can be used in place of refrigerated ravioli but will require a longer cooking time in the sauce until heated through, 6 to 8 minutes. Thawing them slightly before cooking can help decrease the cooking time.

PER SERVING: Calories: 367; Total fat: 15g; Saturated fat: 8g; Sodium: 1,182mg; Carbohydrates: 39g; Fiber: 4g; Protein: 21g; Calcium: 396mg; Potassium: 730mg

SALMON, ARTICHOKE, AND SUN-DRIED TOMATO PASTA SALAD

EXTRA LOW CALORIE

PREP TIME: 5 minutes   **COOK TIME:** 10 minutes
SERVES 4

I refer to this recipe as Pantry Pasta Salad because it's made entirely from staple foods in my home. This option makes a quick lunch when fresh items are limited, and it always leaves leftovers to enjoy another day. Swap the salmon for tuna, shrimp, or grilled chicken. If desired, go with a high-protein or legume-based pasta for added protein and fiber.

8 ounces medium-size pasta, such as penne, gemelli, or fusilli (2 cups dry)

1 (14-ounce) can quartered artichoke hearts, drained

½ cup sun-dried tomatoes, chopped

1 (5-ounce) can or packet salmon

½ cup light Italian dressing, such as Walden Farms

2 tablespoons shredded Parmesan cheese

1. Cook the pasta according to the package directions. Drain and rinse with cold water.

2. Place the cooked pasta in a large bowl. Add the artichoke hearts, sun-dried tomatoes, and salmon. Stir to combine. Add the dressing and sprinkle with the cheese. Toss to coat and serve.

3. Store leftover pasta salad in the refrigerator for up to 3 days.

LOVE YOUR LEFTOVERS: If using leftovers, toss with additional dressing before serving, as the pasta will absorb the liquid. Enjoy straight from the refrigerator or warmed in the microwave.

PER SERVING: Calories: 336; Total fat: 6g; Saturated fat: 1g; Sodium: 484mg; Carbohydrates: 55g; Fiber: 9g; Protein: 18g; Calcium: 70mg; Potassium: 671mg

ONE-POT SHRIMP AND SPINACH PASTA

ONE-POT

PREP TIME: 5 minutes   **COOK TIME:** 20 minutes

SERVES 4

This one-pot meal comes together super quickly and is mostly hands-off. The pasta cooks in broth and tomato sauce to add flavor, eliminating the need to drain and strain. Shrimp and spinach add protein and veggies to this meal and get cooked right in the sauce. Boost your veggies even more by serving this with a side salad.

1 tablespoon olive oil

1 cup chopped onions

3 garlic cloves, minced

1 (28-ounce) can crushed tomatoes

2 cups low-sodium chicken broth

1 tablespoon Italian seasoning

8 ounces medium-size pasta, such as penne, farfalle, or gemelli (2 cups dry)

1 pound shrimp, peeled and deveined, tail-on

4 cups baby spinach

¼ cup grated Parmesan cheese

1. In a large pot, heat the olive oil over medium heat. Add the onions and sauté until translucent, 3 to 5 minutes. Add the garlic and sauté for 30 seconds, until fragrant.

2. Add the crushed tomatoes, broth, Italian seasoning, and pasta. Stir to combine, increase the heat to medium-high, and bring to a boil. Cover, reduce the heat to low, and simmer for 10 minutes, stirring occasionally.

3. Stir in the shrimp and continue cooking, covered, for 3 minutes, until the shrimp is pink and cooked through. Remove from the heat and stir in the spinach and Parmesan cheese.

4. Store leftovers in the refrigerator for up to 4 days.

SIMPLE SWAP: You can replace the shrimp with chicken by adding cooked chicken at the end along with the Parmesan cheese. Feel free to skip the protein to serve as a side dish.

PER SERVING: Calories: 456; Total fat: 8g; Saturated fat: 2g; Sodium: 682mg; Carbohydrates: 62g; Fiber: 7g; Protein: 39g; Calcium: 252mg; Potassium: 1,347mg

PENNE VODKA WITH ARTICHOKES AND ROASTED RED PEPPERS

EXTRA LOW CALORIE

PREP TIME: 5 minutes   **COOK TIME:** 20 minutes
SERVES 4

Vodka sauce is typically a higher-calorie treat due to the use of heavy cream, butter, and lots of cheese. This better-for-you vodka sauce uses Greek yogurt to replace the heavy cream and add protein. You can put this meal together with pantry staples, and it can be done faster than ordering takeout.

8 ounces penne pasta (2 cups dry)

1 tablespoon olive oil

1 shallot, minced

3 garlic cloves, minced

¼ teaspoon red pepper flakes

1 (6-ounce) can tomato paste

¼ cup vodka

¾ cup nonfat plain Greek yogurt

4 tablespoons grated Parmesan cheese, divided

1 (14-ounce) can quartered artichoke hearts, drained

½ cup roasted red pepper strips

¼ cup basil, thinly sliced

1. Cook the pasta according to the package directions. Reserve 2 cups of the pasta water before draining. Set aside.

2. In a large skillet, heat the olive oil over medium heat. Add the shallots and garlic and sauté for 2 to 3 minutes, stirring frequently, until softened.

3. Add the red pepper flakes and tomato paste to the pan and stir to combine. Continue stirring for 5 minutes, until the mixture darkens.

4. Add the vodka and deglaze the pan, using a rubber spatula to scrape up any browned bits. Continue stirring for 2 to 3 minutes, until the mixture thickens.

5. Reduce the heat to low and stir in the Greek yogurt and 2 tablespoons of Parmesan cheese. Add ¼ cup of reserved pasta water and continue adding water, ¼ cup at a time, until your desired consistency is reached.

6. Mix in the pasta to fully coat it with sauce. Add the artichokes, red peppers, basil, and remaining 2 tablespoons of Parmesan cheese, stirring until combined. If the sauce is too thick, stir in additional pasta water.

7. Store leftovers covered in the refrigerator for 3 to 4 days. Add an additional tablespoon of water before reheating.

PER SERVING: Calories: 391; Total fat: 7g; Saturated fat: 2g; Sodium: 200mg; Carbohydrates: 60g; Fiber: 10g; Protein: 17g; Calcium: 151mg; Potassium: 872mg

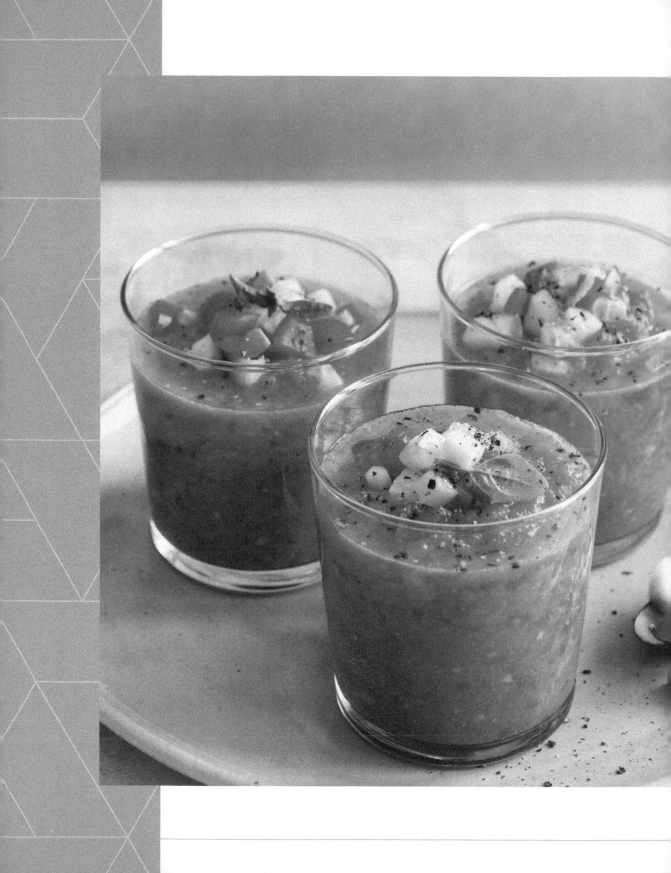

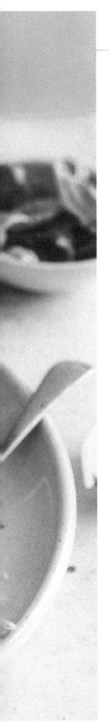

CHAPTER FIVE

Soups and Other Simmerings

Soup is a food that brings up cozy feelings. As you're reading this, words like *comfort*, *warmth*, or *nostalgia* might come to mind. One word I hope you're not thinking is *boring*. The soups in this chapter were created to remind you that soup can be a satisfying meal and not just a side dish or appetizer. These are headliner soups and simmered dishes, many of which are worthy of sharing the spotlight with some warm, crusty bread. Remember—it's all about balance.

GAZPACHO

Gazpacho is a chilled version of tomato soup that tastes refreshing on a hot day. It features lots of summer produce, which is a great way to use in-season vegetables. The best part is that a blender does most of the work, so minimal prep is involved. Add texture to this smooth soup by dicing up some extra tomatoes, watermelon, and cucumber with cilantro for a salsa to serve on top.

1 pound tomatoes (campari, plum, or heirloom), quartered

1 cup cubed seedless watermelon

1 red bell pepper, chopped

½ seedless English cucumber, chopped

1 garlic clove, smashed

2 tablespoons red wine vinegar

2 tablespoons chopped cilantro or parsley

½ jalapeño, seeded and diced (optional)

⅓ cup olive oil

Salt

Freshly ground black pepper

1. In a high-powered blender, combine the tomatoes, watermelon, bell pepper, cucumber, garlic, vinegar, cilantro, and jalapeño (if using). Puree until smooth.

2. While the blender is running, slowly pour in the olive oil until combined. Season with salt and pepper to taste. Divide among four bowls or chill until ready to serve.

3. Store leftover gazpacho in the refrigerator for up to 5 days or freeze for up to 6 months.

COOKING HACK: Gazpacho is typically chilled for a few hours before serving. If you're short on time, you can place serving bowls in the freezer to chill while preparing the soup, then pour the soup into the cold bowls.

PER SERVING: Calories: 208; Total fat: 18g; Saturated fat: 3g; Sodium: 49mg; Carbohydrates: 11g; Fiber: 3g; Protein: 2g; Calcium: 27mg; Potassium: 451mg

TOMATO-BASIL SOUP

EXTRA LOW CALORIE   ONE-POT

PREP TIME: 5 minutes   **COOK TIME:** 25 minutes

SERVES 6

I think there is nothing better on a cold winter day than tomato soup. This Tomato-Basil Soup may take a few more minutes than heating up a canned soup, but the flavor can't be compared—plus there's less sodium in this version. Serve this soup topped with crunchy croutons, pepitas, or Parmesan Crisps (page 148), along with a tasty sandwich or bread for dipping.

2 tablespoons olive oil

1 sweet onion, diced

3 garlic cloves, minced

2 (28-ounce) cans whole peeled tomatoes, with juices

2 cups low-sodium chicken broth

1 tablespoon apple cider vinegar

½ cup chopped basil leaves, plus more for garnish

1. In a large stockpot, heat the oil over medium-high heat. Sauté the onions until translucent and soft, 5 to 7 minutes. Stir in the garlic and sauté for another minute, until fragrant.

2. Add the tomatoes with juices, broth, and vinegar. Bring to a simmer, reduce the heat to medium-low, cover, and continue simmering for 15 minutes, stirring occasionally.

3. Remove the pot from the heat and add the basil.

4. Using an immersion blender, puree the soup until smooth. Alternatively, transfer the liquid to a food processor or blender in small batches to carefully puree. Serve immediately with additional basil for garnish.

5. Store leftover soup in the refrigerator for 5 to 7 days or freeze for up to 6 months.

SIMPLE SWAP: For a creamier soup, add 1 cup low-fat milk before pureeing or top with a dollop of crème fraîche.

PER SERVING: Calories: 116; Total fat: 6g; Saturated fat: 1g; Sodium: 55mg; Carbohydrates: 15g; Fiber: 6g; Protein: 4g; Calcium: 108mg; Potassium: 654mg

PUMPKIN AND PEAR SOUP

5-INGREDIENT   EXTRA LOW CALORIE   ONE-POT
PREP TIME: 5 minutes   **COOK TIME:** 15 minutes
SERVES 4

The traditional version of this soup is made by roasting fresh pumpkin and pears, then simmering and pureeing the mixture. Delicious, but not everybody has time for that. This seasonal fall soup comes together in minutes thanks to canned pumpkin and pears. Look for canned pears that come in their natural juices to reduce added sugars. Top this soup with pepitas or pomegranate seeds for a crunchy texture, and garnish with seasonal herbs such as thyme, sage, or rosemary.

1 (15-ounce) can pumpkin puree

1 (15-ounce) can pears (slices or halves), drained

2 cups low-sodium chicken broth

¼ cup white wine

½ teaspoon ground cinnamon

1. In a medium saucepan, combine the pumpkin and pears. Using an immersion blender, blend the ingredients together until smooth.

2. Place the saucepan over medium heat and add the broth, wine, and cinnamon. Stir to blend, then cover and bring the soup to a boil. Reduce the heat and simmer for 15 minutes, stirring occasionally. Serve immediately.

3. Store leftovers in the refrigerator for 3 to 4 days or freeze for up to 3 months.

COOKING HACK: If you don't have an immersion blender, you can puree the pumpkin and pears in a food processor, then transfer the mixture to the saucepan.

PER SERVING: Calories: 117; Total fat: 1g; Saturated fat: 0g; Sodium: 43mg; Carbohydrates: 24g; Fiber: 6g; Protein: 4g; Calcium: 45mg; Potassium: 433mg

ROSEMARY, PARMESAN, AND CAULIFLOWER SOUP

5-INGREDIENT   EXTRA LOW CALORIE   ONE-POT
PREP TIME: 5 minutes   **COOK TIME:** 25 minutes
SERVES 6

Create a creamy low-calorie cauliflower soup loaded with flavor, thanks to fresh rosemary and Parmesan cheese. Enjoy this soup on its own or paired with a salad, such as Grilled Halloumi Salad (page 46). This soup can be made dairy-free by replacing the Parmesan cheese with nutritional yeast.

1 tablespoon olive oil

½ sweet onion, diced

Salt

Freshly ground black pepper

4 cups cauliflower florets (1 head)

1 (32-ounce) container low-sodium chicken broth

3 rosemary sprigs, plus more for garnish

½ cup shredded Parmesan cheese, plus more for garnish

1. In a large stockpot, heat the oil over medium-high heat. Add the onions, season with salt and pepper, and sauté until translucent and soft, 3 to 5 minutes.

2. Add the cauliflower, broth, and rosemary. Cover, reduce the heat to medium, and simmer for 15 to 20 minutes, until the cauliflower is tender and can be pierced with a fork.

3. Remove the pot from the heat and discard the rosemary sprigs. Using an immersion blender, puree the soup. Alternatively, transfer the mixture in batches to a blender and carefully blend.

4. Stir in the Parmesan cheese until melted. Serve immediately topped with additional rosemary and cheese.

5. Store leftover soup in the refrigerator for up to 5 days or freeze up to 6 months. Reheat on the stovetop.

COOKING HACK: For additional flavor, cook a few strips of bacon in the stockpot first. Remove the bacon to cook the soup in the bacon drippings, then top the finished soup with chopped bacon.

PER SERVING: Calories: 107; Total fat: 6g; Saturated fat: 2g; Sodium: 248mg; Carbohydrates: 9g; Fiber: 2g; Protein: 7g; Calcium: 99mg; Potassium: 399mg

PASTA FAGIOLI WITH ESCAROLE

EXTRA LOW CALORIE   ONE-POT
PREP TIME: 5 minutes   **COOK TIME:** 20 minutes
SERVES 6

This staple Italian "pasta with beans" dish gets a mash-up with another classic soup—escarole and beans—for a hearty meal. The pasta will soak up the liquid over time, so you may want to stir in some additional broth or water before reheating. Soups with pasta don't typically freeze well, as the pasta becomes mushy when defrosted.

---

2 tablespoons olive oil

1 yellow onion, diced

2 medium carrots, peeled and small diced

2 celery stalks, small diced

3 garlic cloves, minced

1 teaspoon Italian seasoning

Salt

Freshly ground black pepper

1 (28-ounce) can crushed tomatoes

2 (15.5-ounce) cans cannellini beans, undrained

2 cups low-sodium chicken broth

1 cup dried ditalini pasta

1 (9-ounce) bag chopped escarole

¼ cup grated Parmesan cheese

Chopped fresh parsley, for garnish (optional)

Red pepper flakes, for garnish (optional)

1. In a large pot, heat the oil over medium-high heat. Add the onion, carrots, and celery and sauté until the vegetables are tender, 5 minutes.

2. Add the garlic and Italian seasoning, season with salt and pepper, and stir for 30 seconds until fragrant.

3. Add the tomatoes, beans, and broth. Cover and bring to a boil.

4. Stir in the ditalini and escarole, reduce the heat to medium, and cook covered for 8 to 10 minutes, until al dente.

5. Remove from the heat and stir in the Parmesan cheese. Serve immediately. Garnish with parsley and red pepper flakes (if using).

6. Store in the refrigerator for up to 5 days.

COOKING HACK: Save and freeze rinds of hard cheeses like Parmesan. Add a rind along with the pasta to provide additional flavor while cooking. Remove the rind before serving.

PER SERVING: Calories: 339; Total fat: 8g; Saturated fat: 2g; Sodium: 409mg; Carbohydrates: 55g; Fiber: 13g; Protein: 17g; Calcium: 206mg; Potassium: 1,197mg

GOLDEN VEGETABLE SOUP WITH ORZO

EXTRA LOW CALORIE   ONE-POT

PREP TIME: 5 minutes   **COOK TIME:** 25 minutes

SERVES 6

Boost your immunity with this antioxidant- and anti-inflammatory–rich soup, thanks to the vegetables, turmeric, and ginger, which may play a role in weight management. If you'd like, add extra antibody-producing protein to this soup with some chopped cooked chicken, chickpeas, or kidney beans.

2 tablespoons olive oil

1 cup yellow onion, diced

1 large carrot, peeled and small diced

2 celery stalks, diced

1 teaspoon ground turmeric

1 teaspoon ground ginger

4 garlic cloves, minced

2 (32-ounce) containers vegetable broth

½ cup dried orzo pasta

1 large zucchini, chopped

Salt

Freshly ground black pepper

Juice of ½ lemon (optional)

1. In a large stockpot, heat the oil over medium-high heat. Add the onion, carrot, and celery and cook until the onion is translucent and the vegetables are tender, 5 to 7 minutes.

2. Add the turmeric, ginger, and garlic, stirring to coat the vegetables. Add the broth, cover, and bring to a boil.

3. Add the orzo and zucchini and boil uncovered for 10 minutes, until the orzo is tender.

4. Season with salt and pepper. Add the lemon juice (if using). Serve immediately.

5. Store leftovers in the refrigerator for 3 to 4 days or freeze for up to 3 months.

COOKING HACK: Using frozen vegetables, including onions, carrots, and zucchini, can cut down on prep time. You can also look in the produce department for prepared *mirepoix*, the French term for diced carrots, celery, and onions, which serves as the base for many soups.

PER SERVING: Calories: 103; Total fat: 5g; Saturated fat: 1g; Sodium: 45mg; Carbohydrates: 13g; Fiber: 2g; Protein: 2g; Calcium: 28mg; Potassium: 275mg

CHICKEN TOMATILLO SOUP

EXTRA LOW CALORIE   ONE-POT
PREP TIME: 5 minutes   **COOK TIME:** 15 minutes
SERVES 4

Tomatillos look like unripe tomatoes with a husk. They have a tangy, acidic flavor, which makes them popular for soups, salsas, and sauces. Tomatillo soup usually involves roasting the tomatillos first, but this quick version uses canned tomatillos for easy blending. Look for canned tomatillos in the international aisle of your grocery store.

2 tablespoons olive oil

1 sweet onion, diced

3 garlic cloves, minced

1 (4-ounce) can diced green chiles

1 jalapeño, seeded and minced

½ tablespoon cumin

½ tablespoon ground coriander

1 teaspoon chili powder

1 (28-ounce) can tomatillos, drained

1 (32-ounce) container chicken stock

2 cups cooked chicken

Juice of ½ lime

1. In a large stockpot, heat the oil over medium-high heat. Sauté the onion and garlic until the onion is translucent, 3 minutes.

2. Add the chiles, jalapeño, cumin, coriander, and chili powder, stirring to coat. Add the tomatillos and stock. Bring to a boil, cover, reduce the heat, and simmer for 10 minutes.

3. Remove the stockpot from the heat. Using an immersion blender, puree the mixture until smooth (or transfer in small batches to a blender to carefully puree). Stir in the chicken and lime juice.

4. Store leftovers in the refrigerator for up to 4 days or freeze for up to 3 months.

SERVING SUGGESTION: Garnish this soup with additional slices of jalapeños, a lime wedge, avocado slices, chopped cilantro, or queso fresco crumbles.

PER SERVING: Calories: 250; Total fat: 11g; Saturated fat: 2g; Sodium: 631mg; Carbohydrates: 16g; Fiber: 5g; Protein: 23g; Calcium: 116mg; Potassium: 739mg

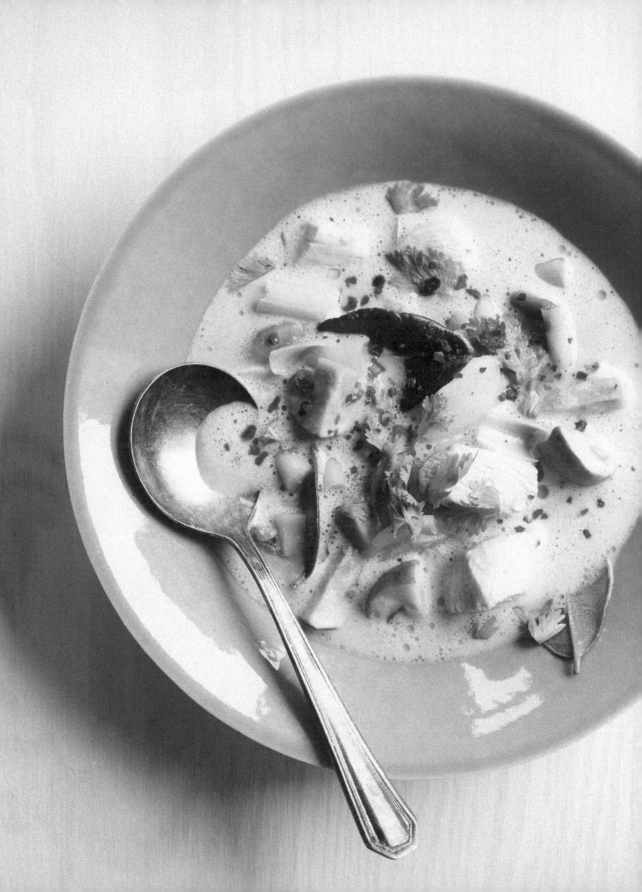

COCONUT CHICKEN SOUP

EXTRA LOW CALORIE   ONE-POT
PREP TIME: 5 minutes   **COOK TIME:** 20 minutes
SERVES 6

Create your own homemade version of *tom kha gai*, a traditional spicy-sour Thai soup made with coconut milk and chicken. By using a light coconut milk, you'll reduce the saturated fat content in an otherwise low-calorie soup that doubles as a meal.

2 tablespoons canola oil

1 (3.5-ounce) container sliced shiitake mushrooms

1 tablespoon grated fresh ginger, or 1 teaspoon ground ginger

6 cups low-sodium chicken broth

1 (14-ounce) can light coconut milk

1 tablespoon fish sauce

1 fresh lemongrass stalk, cut into 1-inch pieces (optional)

1 pound boneless, skinless chicken thighs, cut into 1-inch pieces

Juice of 1 lime

Chopped basil, for garnish

Chopped cilantro, for garnish

Chili oil, for garnish

1. In a large stockpot, heat the oil over medium-high heat. Add the mushrooms and sauté until softened, 2 minutes. Add the ginger and stir to coat the mushrooms, cooking for 2 minutes, until fragrant.

2. Stir in the broth, coconut milk, fish sauce, and lemongrass (if using). Cover and bring to a boil.

3. Add the chicken, reduce the heat to a simmer, cover, and simmer for 15 minutes, until the chicken is cooked through.

4. Using a skimmer or slotted spoon, remove the lemongrass. Stir in the lime juice, garnish the bowls with the chopped basil, cilantro, and chili oil and serve.

5. Store leftovers in the refrigerator for up to 5 days or freeze for up to 3 months.

COOKING HACK: Use a citrus press juicer to add fresh lime juice directly into the soup. Make sure the flat side of the sliced half of the lime is facing down before squeezing.

PER SERVING: Calories: 295; Total fat: 21g; Saturated fat: 12g; Sodium: 389mg; Carbohydrates: 8g; Fiber: 2g; Protein: 21g; Calcium: 26mg; Potassium: 592mg

PORK HOT AND SOUR SOUP

EXTRA LOW CALORIE   ONE-POT
PREP TIME: 10 minutes   **COOK TIME:** 15 minutes
SERVES 6

Warm up on a cold day with a version of this Chinese restaurant classic also known as "peppered vinegar soup." This recipe gets its spice from gochujang paste, a savory, sweet, and spicy red chili paste popular in Korean dishes. You'll find gochujang paste in the international aisle of most grocery stores. Omit the pork for a meatless version.

2 tablespoons canola oil

8 ounces thin boneless pork chops, cut into ¼-inch strips

8 ounces sliced shiitake or cremini mushrooms

2 teaspoons ground ginger

1 teaspoon gochujang paste

6 cups low-sodium chicken broth

½ cup low-sodium soy sauce

⅓ cup rice wine vinegar

3 tablespoons cornstarch

¼ cup water

2 large eggs, beaten

4 ounces firm tofu, cut into ½-inch cubes

3 scallions, sliced

1 teaspoon sesame oil

⅛ teaspoon white pepper or freshly ground black pepper

1. In a large stockpot, heat the oil over high heat. Add the pork and mushrooms and cook, stirring frequently, until the pork is browned and cooked through, 2 to 3 minutes. Add the ginger and gochujang, stirring to coat the pork and mushrooms.

2. Add the broth, soy sauce, and rice wine vinegar to the pot and bring to a simmer.

3. In a small bowl, whisk together the cornstarch and water. Stir the cornstarch mixture into the broth and allow it to thicken for 1 minute.

4. While constantly stirring the broth in a circular motion, slowly pour in the beaten eggs to create ribbons (see Technique Trick). Add the tofu, scallions, sesame oil, and pepper, stirring to combine. Remove from the heat and serve immediately.

5. Store leftovers in the refrigerator for up to 3 days or freeze for up to 3 months. If you plan to freeze this soup, wait to add the tofu until you're ready to serve.

TECHNIQUE TRICK: Beat the eggs together in a liquid measuring cup to help control pouring the eggs into the soup.

PER SERVING: Calories: 228; Total fat: 12g; Saturated fat: 2g; Sodium: 886mg; Carbohydrates: 11g; Fiber: 1g; Protein: 22g; Calcium: 164mg; Potassium: 649mg

TORTELLINI, KALE, AND SAUSAGE SOUP

ONE-POT

PREP TIME: 5 minutes   **COOK TIME:** 25 minutes

SERVES 4

This soup comes together for a quick meal thanks to frozen cheese-filled tortellini. The Italian-seasoned sausage provides wonderful flavor to the soup as it simmers. If you're looking for a spicier version, swap in hot Italian sausage and top with red pepper flakes.

1 tablespoon olive oil

1 pound sweet Italian sausage, casings removed

1 yellow onion, diced

4 garlic cloves, minced

1 (32-ounce) container low-sodium chicken broth

2 cups water

2 bay leaves

¼ teaspoon salt

¼ teaspoon freshly ground black pepper

3 cups chopped kale

2 cups frozen cheese-filled tortellini

Red pepper flakes, for garnish (optional)

Parmesan cheese, for garnish (optional)

1. In a large pot, heat the oil over medium-high heat. Add the sausage, onion, and garlic. Sauté and break up the sausage until browned and cooked through, 5 minutes.

2. Add the broth, water, bay leaves, salt, and pepper. Cover and bring to a boil, then reduce the heat and simmer for 15 minutes.

3. Discard the bay leaves. Stir in the kale and tortellini. Simmer uncovered for 2 to 3 minutes, until the pasta is cooked through and the kale starts to wilt. Serve immediately, garnished with red pepper flakes or Parmesan cheese (if using).

4. Store leftover soup in the refrigerator for up to 5 days or freeze without the tortellini. Add the tortellini when reheating.

COOKING HACK: Look for ground sweet or spicy Italian sausage meat to skip the step of removing the casings.

PER SERVING: Calories: 424; Total fat: 18g; Saturated fat: 7g; Sodium: 821mg; Carbohydrates: 35g; Fiber: 2g; Protein: 31g; Calcium: 150mg; Potassium: 586mg

BEEF BARLEY SOUP

EXTRA LOW CALORIE   ONE-POT
PREP TIME: 5 minutes   **COOK TIME:** 25 minutes
SERVES 6

Barley is a whole grain that typically needs an hour to cook, which is why beef barley soup usually takes longer to create. This version uses quick-cooking barley, which cooks in under 15 minutes, along with frozen vegetables and flavorful stock, to create a delicious hearty soup in half the time.

2 tablespoons olive oil, divided

8 ounces sirloin steak, cut into bite-size pieces

Salt

Freshly ground black pepper

1 cup frozen chopped onions

1 celery stalk, small diced

2 tablespoons tomato paste

1 teaspoon dried thyme

¼ cup red wine

1 cup frozen peas and carrots

¾ cup quick-cooking barley

1 (32-ounce) container beef stock or bone broth

1 cup water

1. In a large stockpot, heat 1 tablespoon of oil over medium-high heat. Add the steak, season with salt and pepper, and cook until browned, stirring frequently, 3 to 5 minutes. Transfer to a bowl along with any juices.

2. In the same large stockpot, heat the remaining 1 tablespoon of oil. Sauté the onion and celery until softened, 2 minutes.

3. Add the tomato paste and thyme, stirring to coat, and cook until the vegetables are browned, 2 to 3 minutes. Add the wine to deglaze the pan, using a spatula to scrape up any browned bits.

4. Add the peas and carrots, barley, stock, and water. Season with additional salt and pepper.

5. Bring the soup to a simmer, then cover, reduce the heat to medium-low, and continue to simmer for 15 minutes, or until the barley is tender.

6. Return the beef and juices to the pot and heat for an additional 1 to 2 minutes. Remove and serve immediately.

7. Store leftover soup in the refrigerator for 3 to 4 days or freeze for up to 3 months.

PER SERVING: Calories: 252; Total fat: 9g; Saturated fat: 2g; Sodium: 498mg; Carbohydrates: 26g; Fiber: 5g; Protein: 15g; Calcium: 38mg; Potassium: 437mg

TURKEY CHILI

ONE-POT
PREP TIME: 5 minutes   **COOK TIME:** 25 minutes
SERVES 4

This is football tailgating food at its finest. Warm up before kickoff with a hot bowl of turkey chili, even if you're just watching at home. This chili can be enjoyed on its own or as a topping for nachos or baked potatoes. You can even use this chili as a filling for Turkey Taco–Stuffed Sweet Potatoes (page 66).

1 tablespoon olive oil

1 cup chopped sweet onions

1 tablespoon minced garlic

½ yellow bell pepper, diced

1 pound ground turkey

1 tablespoon chili powder

1 tablespoon ground cumin

1 (28-ounce) can crushed tomatoes

1 (15.5-ounce) can kidney beans, drained and rinsed

⅔ cup low-sodium chicken stock

½ tablespoon kosher salt

1 teaspoon hot sauce (optional)

Shredded cheddar cheese, for garnish

1. In a large stockpot, heat the oil over medium-high heat. Sauté the onions, garlic, and bell pepper until the onions are translucent, 3 to 5 minutes.

2. Add the ground turkey, chili powder, and cumin. Using a wooden spoon, break up the meat while stirring. Cook until browned, 3 to 5 minutes.

3. Stir in the tomatoes, beans, stock, salt, and hot sauce (if using). Bring to a boil, then reduce the heat to medium-low, cover, and simmer for 15 minutes. Serve immediately. Top with shredded cheese when serving.

4. Store leftover chili in the refrigerator for up to 3 days or freeze for 4 to 6 months.

SIMPLE SWAP: Amp up the flavor of your chili by swapping ⅓ cup chicken stock for ⅓ cup beer, such as a lager or stout.

PER SERVING: Calories: 414; Total fat: 18g; Saturated fat: 6g; Sodium: 796mg; Carbohydrates: 30g; Fiber: 10g; Protein: 35g; Calcium: 244mg; Potassium: 1,144mg

WHITE BEAN CHICKEN CHILI

PREP TIME: 5 minutes **COOK TIME:** 25 minutes
SERVES 4

Change up your usual chili for an alternative version starring white beans that provide a creamy texture. This protein-rich chili can be enjoyed on its own or served with Jalapeño-Cheddar Corn Muffins (page 62) for dipping.

2 (15.5-ounce) cans white beans, drained and rinsed, divided

2 cups low-sodium chicken stock, divided

1 tablespoon olive oil

1 sweet onion, diced

3 garlic cloves, minced

1 tablespoon chili powder

½ tablespoon ground cumin

2 (4-ounce) cans diced green chiles

2 cups shredded cooked chicken

1 cup frozen corn

Juice of 1 lime

2 tablespoons chopped cilantro

Salt

Freshly ground black pepper

1. In a food processor or blender, puree 1 can of drained beans with ¼ cup of stock. Set aside.

2. In a large stockpot, heat the oil over medium-high heat. Sauté the onion and garlic in the stockpot until translucent, 3 to 5 minutes.

3. Add the chili powder and cumin and stir until fragrant and combined. Stir in the chiles and remaining 1 can of beans to coat. Add the bean puree, remaining 1¾ cups of stock, chicken, and corn. Cover and simmer for 15 minutes.

4. Stir in the lime juice and cilantro. Season with salt and pepper and serve. The chili will continue to thicken as it cools.

5. Store leftovers in the refrigerator for up to 4 days or freeze for up to 3 months.

SERVING SUGGESTION: Garnish with additional cilantro, jalapeño slices, a lime wedge, avocado slices, or pepper Jack cheese.

PER SERVING: Calories: 441; Total fat: 8g; Saturated fat: 2g; Sodium: 188mg; Carbohydrates: 58g; Fiber: 13g; Protein: 37g; Calcium: 179mg; Potassium: 1,459mg

CHICKEN AND DUMPLINGS

EXTRA LOW CALORIE   ONE-POT
PREP TIME: 5 minutes   **COOK TIME:** 15 minutes
SERVES 6

I love a good chicken and dumplings stew, but sometimes it can be so heavy that it leaves me feeling weighted down. This lightened-up version cuts back on the heavy cream and butter and comes together super quickly by using frozen vegetables and gnocchi for dumplings.

1 (14.5-ounce) can low-sodium chicken broth

1 (12-ounce) package frozen mixed vegetables

1 cup frozen chopped onions

½ cup water

½ teaspoon dried oregano

⅛ teaspoon garlic powder

⅛ teaspoon freshly ground black pepper

1 bay leaf

1 cup low-fat milk

½ cup all-purpose flour

2 cups cooked chicken, cubed

1 (16-ounce) package refrigerated potato gnocchi

1. In a large stockpot over high heat, add the broth, frozen vegetables, onions, water, oregano, garlic powder, pepper, and bay leaf. Bring to a boil.

2. In a small bowl, whisk together the milk and flour until smooth.

3. Stir the milk-and-flour mixture into the boiling mixture. Add the chicken and stir until thickened and bubbly, 1 to 2 minutes. Cover and reduce the heat to simmer for 10 minutes. The volume should double in this time.

4. Remove the pot from the heat. Discard the bay leaf, stir in the gnocchi, and let it sit for 1 minute to heat the gnocchi. Serve immediately.

5. Store leftovers in the refrigerator for up to 5 days. Add some milk and broth before reheating to thin it a bit.

COOKING HACK: A store-bought rotisserie chicken can be used in any recipe that calls for cooked chicken. Remove the meat and store in the refrigerator until needed.

PER SERVING: Calories: 290; Total fat: 8g; Saturated fat: 4g; Sodium: 304mg; Carbohydrates: 34g; Fiber: 4g; Protein: 20g; Calcium: 97mg; Potassium: 487mg

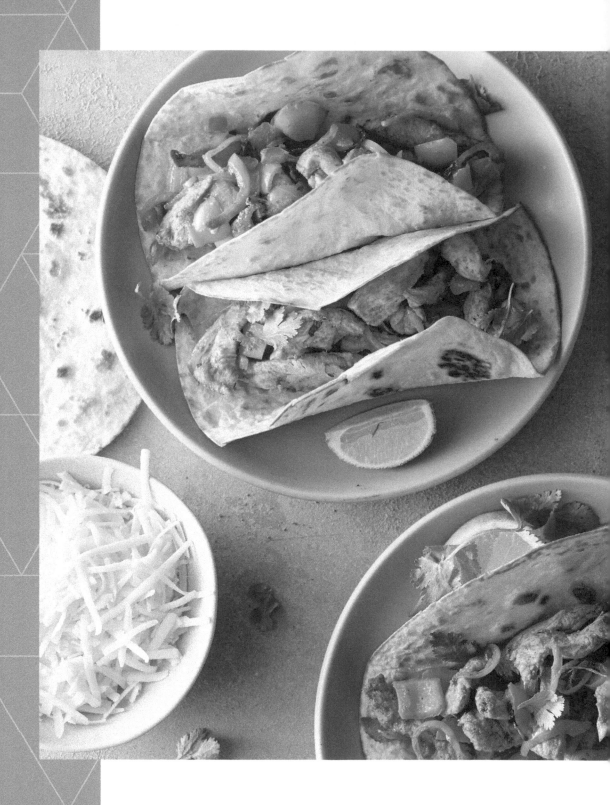

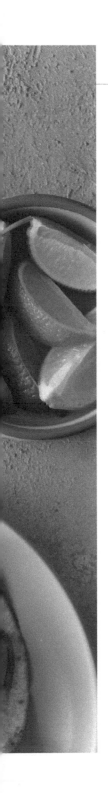

CHAPTER SIX

Seafood and Poultry

The top protein in my home is seafood. I'm lucky enough to live by the water, and there are so many varieties of seafood that keep meals interesting. I hope to introduce you to new preparation methods and ways to enjoy it. Like seafood, chicken also offers tons of versatility for meals. In fact, chicken and seafood can be swapped in many of the recipes in this chapter. Make sure to maximize leftovers for busy weeks!

SHRIMP RAMEN

EXTRA LOW CALORIE   ONE-POT
PREP TIME: 5 minutes   **COOK TIME:** 15 minutes
SERVES 4

Ramen is my go-to comfort food when I'm not feeling well. The noodles and spicy broth from this recipe always cheer me up; plus, the veggies and protein help boost immunity. Create your own comforting lower-sodium ramen at home faster than you can order takeout.

1 tablespoon avocado oil

1 (8-ounce) container sliced mushrooms

1 cup shredded carrots

4 garlic cloves, minced

1 teaspoon red pepper flakes

2 tablespoons white miso paste

2 (32-ounce) containers vegetable broth

1 tablespoon low-sodium soy sauce

1 tablespoon sesame oil

2 (3-ounce) packages ramen noodles, seasoning packets discarded

1 pound medium shrimp, peeled and deveined

1. In a large stockpot over medium-high heat, heat the avocado oil. Add the mushrooms and carrots and sauté until softened, 3 to 5 minutes.

2. Add the garlic and red pepper flakes and sauté for 30 seconds until fragrant. Stir the miso paste into the mixture. Add the broth, soy sauce, and sesame oil. Cover the pot and bring to a boil, 5 minutes.

3. Once the broth is boiling, add the ramen noodles and shrimp. Stir, then cover and cook for 3 minutes, until the shrimp is pink and cooked through and the noodles are tender.

4. Spoon the soup into four bowls and garnish with your desired toppings (see Serving Suggestion).

5. Store leftover ramen in the refrigerator for up to 5 days.

SERVING SUGGESTION: Top the ramen with a soft-boiled egg cut in half. See page 41 for how to soft-boil an egg. Garnish with sliced scallions, chopped cilantro, or additional vegetables.

PER SERVING: Calories: 278; Total fat: 12g; Saturated fat: 2g; Sodium: 421mg; Carbohydrates: 16g; Fiber: 2g; Protein: 29g; Calcium: 103mg; Potassium: 857mg

SHRIMP PICCATA

ONE-POT

PREP TIME: 5 minutes   **COOK TIME:** 15 minutes

SERVES 4

Making this classic Italian meal at home saves you time, money, and calories. Flavors of tart lemon, sweet shallot, and salty capers come together beautifully in this saucy dish. You can also create this recipe with any flaky white fish or thin chicken breasts.

2 tablespoons olive oil

1½ pounds jumbo shrimp, deveined, tail-on

Salt

Freshly ground black pepper

½ cup all-purpose flour

6 tablespoons (¾ stick) unsalted butter, divided

2 tablespoons minced shallot

½ cup dry white wine

½ cup vegetable broth

Juice of 1½ lemons

2 tablespoons capers, drained

2 tablespoons chopped fresh parsley

1. Preheat a large nonstick skillet over medium heat with the olive oil.

2. Season the shrimp with salt and pepper. In a large zip-top bag, combine the flour and shrimp and shake to dredge them.

3. Shake off any excess flour and place the shrimp in the skillet. Cook for 2 minutes per side, until lightly browned. Transfer the cooked shrimp to a plate. Set aside.

4. Melt 2 tablespoons of butter in the skillet. Add the shallot and cook until soft, 30 seconds. Add the wine, broth, and lemon juice. Increase the heat to medium-high and cook for 5 minutes, until the liquid is thickened and slightly reduced.

5. Reduce the heat to low and stir in the remaining 4 tablespoons of butter, capers, and parsley until the butter is melted. Return the shrimp to the pan and toss in the sauce until coated.

6. Store leftover shrimp in the refrigerator for up to 3 days.

SERVING SUGGESTION: Pair with Rosemary-Parmesan Smashed Potatoes (page 135) and Roasted Shaved Brussels Sprouts (page 131) or serve over pasta or zoodles.

PER SERVING: Calories: 448; Total fat: 25g; Saturated fat: 12g; Sodium: 348mg; Carbohydrates: 15g; Fiber: 1g; Protein: 36g; Calcium: 126mg; Potassium: 539mg

PESCATARIAN SURF AND TURF (SHRIMP WITH CAULIFLOWER STEAKS)

5-INGREDIENT   EXTRA LOW CALORIE   ONE-POT
PREP TIME: 10 minutes   **COOK TIME:** 10 minutes
SERVES 4

This meal comes from a different turf—the ground! Cauliflower is used to create hearty steaks served up with shellfish. Everything gets cooked on the grill or a grill pan for a simple no-fuss meal. Serve this along with a salad, such as the Watermelon, Tomato, Cucumber, Feta, and Mint Salad (page 42) for a complete meal loaded with fruits and veggies.

2 heads cauliflower

½ cup olive oil, plus
   1 tablespoon

1 tablespoon steak seasoning

1 pound medium shrimp,
   deveined, tail-on

1 teaspoon freshly ground
   black pepper

Juice of 1 lemon

1. Preheat a grill or grill pan over medium-high heat.

2. Slice the bottoms of the cauliflower heads to remove the stem and leaves. Place the flat bottom on a cutting board and slice a quarter off each end. Slice the remainder of the cauliflower in half to create 2 "steaks," 1 to 1½ inches thick.

3. In a small bowl, combine ½ cup of olive oil with the steak seasoning. Brush the oil mixture all over the cauliflower steaks to coat.

4. In a medium bowl or zip-top bag, combine the shrimp with the remaining 1 tablespoon of olive oil and the black pepper. If desired, place the shrimp on skewers.

5. Place the cauliflower on the grill to cook for 3 to 5 minutes per side, until browned and tender. While turning the cauliflower, place the shrimp on the grill to cook for 2 minutes per side, until pink. Remove the cauliflower and shrimp from the grill. Drizzle lemon juice over the shrimp.

6. Store leftover cauliflower and shrimp in the refrigerator for up to 2 days.

LOVE YOUR LEFTOVERS: Save the remaining ends of the cauliflower to serve with another meal or toss into salads or bowls, such as Pesto Grain Bowl with Chickpeas (page 50).

PER SERVING: Calories: 355; Total fat: 29g; Saturated fat: 4g; Sodium: 682mg; Carbohydrates: 8g; Fiber: 3g; Protein: 18g; Calcium: 91mg; Potassium: 537mg

HONEY-SOY FISH TACOS WITH MANDARIN SLAW

EXTRA LOW CALORIE

PREP TIME: 15 minutes   **COOK TIME:** 5 minutes
SERVES 3

Give your Taco Tuesday a makeover with fish tacos. These fish tacos come together quickly and give your plate a pop of color, thanks to the fruits and veggies in the slaw. Loaded with lean protein and fiber, they prove you can lose weight while still enjoying tacos.

¼ cup low-sodium soy sauce

3 tablespoons honey

2 tablespoons sesame oil

½ teaspoon ground ginger

3 tablespoons sliced scallions, divided

1 pound flaky white fish, such as tilapia or cod

2 cups coleslaw mix, or 1 cup coleslaw mix and 1 cup shredded red cabbage

½ cup mandarin oranges, drained and cut in half

6 (6-inch) corn tortillas, warmed

1. Preheat the oven broiler on high (550°F). Line a sheet pan with nonstick aluminum foil.

2. In a small bowl, whisk together the soy sauce, honey, sesame oil, ginger, and 2 tablespoons of scallions to create the marinade.

3. In a large zip-top bag, combine the fish and add ½ cup of the marinade. Place the bag of fish in the refrigerator to marinate for 10 minutes.

4. In a medium bowl, combine the coleslaw mix, mandarin oranges, and remaining 1 tablespoon of scallions. Add the remaining marinade and stir to combine.

5. Place the marinated fish on the prepared sheet pan and brush on additional marinade from the zip-top bag. Discard remaining marinade. Broil the fish for 3 minutes per side, until browned on top.

6. Assemble the tacos with the corn tortillas, the fish, and the slaw mixture. Garnish with your desired toppings (see Serving Suggestion).

7. Store any leftover fish and slaw separately in sealed containers in the refrigerator for up to 3 days.

SERVING SUGGESTION: Top these tacos with thinly sliced mini sweet bell peppers, sliced almonds, chopped cilantro, or sesame seeds. Enjoy any leftover slaw as a side dish.

PER SERVING: Calories: 316; Total fat: 6g; Saturated fat: 1g; Sodium: 823mg; Carbohydrates: 38g; Fiber: 5g; Protein: 27g; Calcium: 117mg; Potassium: 658mg

FISH EN PAPILLOTE

EXTRA LOW CALORIE   ONE-POT
PREP TIME: 10 minutes   COOK TIME: 15 minutes
SERVES 4

Cooking "en papillote" means cooking in paper. This popular French technique may sound fancy, but it's a quick and simple way to cook a meal. Cooking fish and vegetables in parchment paper with seasonings and aromatics steams the ingredients while also creating portion-controlled servings.

1 bunch asparagus, woody ends removed

1½ pounds codfish (or any flaky white fish), cut into 4 fillets

Salt

Freshly ground black pepper

8 thyme sprigs

2 lemons, sliced

1 medium shallot, sliced

4 tablespoons (½ stick) unsalted butter

1 pint grape tomatoes, halved

2 tablespoons olive oil

1. Preheat the oven to 425°F. Line a sheet pan with foil.

2. Tear off 4 squares of parchment paper, about 12 inches in length. Divide the asparagus between the parchment squares and place in a single layer in the middle of the paper.

3. Season the fish on both sides with salt and pepper and place on top of the asparagus. Place 2 thyme sprigs on top of each piece of fish, then alternate lemon and shallot slices over the thyme. Top the lemon and shallots with 3 or 4 slices of butter.

4. Place the tomato halves next to the asparagus. Drizzle the olive oil over the fish and vegetables and season with additional salt and pepper.

5. Create the parchment packet by bringing the two long ends together above a fillet, then folding and creasing three times to seal. Fold the short ends under the packet. Place the packets on the prepared sheet pan and bake for 12 to 15 minutes, until cooked through (internal temperature of 145°F).

6. Carefully open the packets, discard the thyme, lemon, and shallots, and enjoy.

SERVING SUGGESTION: Serve along with Quinoa with Toasted Pine Nuts and Tomato (page 133).

PER SERVING: Calories: 295; Total fat: 19g; Saturated fat: 8g; Sodium: 559mg; Carbohydrates: 3g; Fiber: 2g; Protein: 27g; Calcium: 32mg; Potassium: 588mg

TILAPIA OREGANATA

EXTRA LOW CALORIE   ONE-POT
PREP TIME: 5 minutes   **COOK TIME:** 15 minutes
SERVES 4

Oreganata style uses a mixture of bread crumbs, oregano, and either butter or oil. It provides a crunchy topping for fish, with a texture that's surprisingly light. This recipe is a perfect way to introduce more seafood into your diet, because it has tons of flavor without a lot of work. This dish is such a hit that it's my husband's go-to when he makes me a fancy dinner.

4 (4-ounce) tilapia fillets (or any white flaky fish)

Zest and juice of 1 lemon, divided

Salt

Freshly ground black pepper

½ cup panko bread crumbs

2 tablespoons seasoned bread crumbs

2 tablespoons dried oregano

2 tablespoons olive oil

½ teaspoon garlic salt

Nonstick cooking spray

1. Preheat the oven to 425°F and line a sheet pan with non-stick aluminum foil.

2. Place the tilapia fillets on the prepared sheet pan and drizzle with 1 tablespoon of lemon juice. Season with salt and pepper.

3. In a small bowl, combine the panko, seasoned bread crumbs, oregano, lemon zest, remaining lemon juice, olive oil, and garlic salt. Stir until combined.

4. Rub the mixture on top of the tilapia fillets. Use your hands or the back of a spoon to gently press the mixture onto the fillets. Spray the fillets with cooking spray and bake for 10 to 15 minutes, until the tops are golden and crispy and the fish is cooked through (internal temperature of 145°F).

5. Store leftovers in the refrigerator for up to 3 days.

SERVING SUGGESTION: Pair this dish with Spicy Garlicky Zoodles (page 129) or the alternative lemon-herb swap. The bread crumbs on top of the tilapia reduce the need for an additional carb.

PER SERVING: Calories: 203; Total fat: 9g; Saturated fat: 2g; Sodium: 148mg; Carbohydrates: 7g; Fiber: 1g; Protein: 24g; Calcium: 49mg; Potassium: 388mg

SEARED TUNA SLIDERS WITH CILANTRO-LIME SLAW

PREP TIME: 10 minutes   **COOK TIME:** 5 minutes
SERVES 4

This isn't your basic backyard barbecue burger. These omega-3 loaded sliders pack a punch of sweet and spicy. If you like spicier foods, add sliced jalapeños. If you prefer no spice, swap the Cajun seasoning for simple salt and pepper. Pan-sear or grill the tuna.

Nonstick cooking spray

2 pounds fresh or thawed frozen yellowfin or ahi tuna steaks

2 tablespoons Cajun or blackening seasoning

2 cups coleslaw mix

½ cup olive oil mayonnaise

Juice of ½ lime

2 tablespoons chopped cilantro

1 avocado, peeled, pitted, and mashed, or premade guacamole

8 toasted slider buns, cut in half horizontally

1 mango, peeled and sliced

1. Heat a large nonstick skillet over high heat. Spray with cooking spray.

2. Cut the tuna into 8 slider-size pieces, about 2½ inches wide. Season with the Cajun seasoning. Let the tuna sit while preparing the slaw.

3. In a medium bowl, stir together the coleslaw mix, mayonnaise, lime juice, and cilantro. Set aside.

4. Sear the tuna in the heated skillet for 90 seconds per side. The inside will still be rare. Cook for an additional 30 to 60 seconds if you prefer a more cooked through tuna. Immediately remove the seared tuna from the skillet.

5. Assemble the sliders by spreading the mashed avocado on the bottom buns. Top with the seared tuna, mango slices, and coleslaw.

6. Store any leftover tuna in a sealed container in the refrigerator for up to 5 days. Assemble on buns just before serving.

LOVE YOUR LEFTOVERS: Use leftover seared tuna on top of salads, such as Kale Caesar Salad (page 41) or in bowls, such as in place of cooked salmon in the Salmon Teriyaki Power Bowl (page 54).

PER SERVING: Calories: 654; Total fat: 24g; Saturated fat: 4g; Sodium: 644mg; Carbohydrates: 47g; Fiber: 8g; Protein: 62g; Calcium: 144mg; Potassium: 1,576mg

SWEET AND SPICY SALMON

5-INGREDIENT   EXTRA LOW CALORIE   ONE-POT
PREP TIME: 5 minutes   **COOK TIME:** 15 minutes
SERVES 4

This crowd-pleasing salmon is a great way to serve heart-healthy seafood. The delicious brown sugar and spices come together and complement the fish when they caramelize. This fish can also be served on top of a salad or bowl, such as the Salmon Teriyaki Power Bowl (page 54).

4 (6-ounce) salmon fillets, skin-on

2 tablespoons brown sugar

½ tablespoon sea salt

1 teaspoon chili powder

1 teaspoon ground cumin

¼ teaspoon freshly ground black pepper

1. Preheat the oven to 425ºF. Line a sheet pan with nonstick aluminum foil.

2. Place the salmon, skin-side down, on the prepared sheet pan.

3. In a small bowl, mix together the brown sugar, sea salt, chili powder, cumin, and black pepper.

4. Rub the brown sugar mixture on top of the salmon, using your hands or the back of a spoon to press the mixture into the salmon.

5. Bake the salmon for 10 minutes. Remove from the oven and turn on the broiler to high (550ºF). Place the salmon on the top rack of the oven under the broiler for 2 to 3 minutes, until the topping is caramelized.

SERVING SUGGESTION: Serve this dish with grains and a vegetable, such as Roasted Shaved Brussels Sprouts (page 131) or steamed asparagus drizzled with Sesame, Miso, and Ginger Dressing (page 139).

PER SERVING: Calories: 263; Total fat: 11g; Saturated fat: 2g; Sodium: 532mg; Carbohydrates: 5g; Fiber: 0g; Protein: 34g; Calcium: 32mg; Potassium: 863mg

GRILLED CHICKEN THIGHS SANDWICH

5-INGREDIENT   ONE-POT

PREP TIME: 10 minutes   **COOK TIME:** 10 minutes

SERVES 4

Whether it's a summertime barbecue, football tailgate, or weekday meal, these grilled chicken sandwiches deliver the sweetness with barbecue sauce and grilled pineapple. Store-bought barbecue sauce (look for low-sugar options, such as Stubb's Original) and presliced pineapple make this meal happen in minutes. No grill? No worries. The chicken and pineapple can be cooked indoors on a grill pan or in the broiler.

1 pound boneless, skinless chicken thighs

½ cup barbecue sauce, plus more for serving if desired

4 pineapple rings, cut into ¼-inch-thick slices

1 avocado, peeled, pitted, and sliced or mashed

4 kaiser rolls

1. Preheat the grill to medium heat (or a grill pan over medium-high heat).

2. Combine the chicken and barbecue sauce in a large zip-top bag. Marinate for 10 minutes in the refrigerator.

3. Transfer the marinated chicken to lie flat on the grill or grill pan and reserve the remaining sauce. Cook for 4 to 5 minutes, until browned. Flip the chicken, brush the remaining reserved sauce over top, and add the pineapple rings to the grill. Discard any remaining sauce.

4. Cook the chicken for an additional 4 to 5 minutes, until browned and cooked through (internal temperature of 165°F). Grill the pineapple for 2 to 3 minutes per side, until browned.

5. Assemble the sandwiches by placing a chicken thigh, a pineapple ring, and avocado on a roll. Top with additional barbecue sauce if desired.

6. Store any leftover grilled chicken in the refrigerator for up to 5 days.

SERVING SUGGESTION: Serve these sandwiches with a side of grilled veggies or a salad such as Beet, Goat Cheese, and Pistachio Salad (page 43).

PER SERVING: Calories: 474; Total fat: 15g; Saturated fat: 3g; Sodium: 789mg; Carbohydrates: 56g; Fiber: 5g; Protein: 29g; Calcium: 86mg; Potassium: 720mg

CHICKEN AND BLACK BEAN QUESADILLAS

EXTRA LOW CALORIE

PREP TIME: 5 minutes   **COOK TIME:** 15 minutes

SERVES 8

My husband and I are big sports fans and love going to sports bars to watch games. However, bar food can get costly with calories, especially when paired with a few beers. Make your own bar eats at home to enjoy as a snack, quick lunch, or party appetizer, like these homemade quesadillas.

1 pound thin sliced boneless, skinless chicken breasts or thighs

1 tablespoon avocado oil

1 tablespoon fajita or taco seasoning

1 (15.5-ounce) can black beans, drained and rinsed

1 (10-ounce) can fire-roasted diced tomatoes with chiles, drained

2 cups shredded cheddar Jack cheese

4 (10-inch) tortillas

1. Preheat the oven broiler on high and line a sheet pan with nonstick aluminum foil.

2. Season the chicken with the oil and fajita seasoning. Broil for 4 minutes per side until browned. Remove from the broiler and let rest for 2 minutes to cool. Keep the broiler on.

3. In a large bowl, combine the black beans with the tomatoes and chiles. Dice the chicken and combine it with the beans and tomatoes.

4. Spread ¼ cup of cheese on half a tortilla, top with filling, and place another ¼ cup of cheese on top. Fold over the tortilla into a half-circle and place on the prepared sheet pan. Repeat with the remaining tortillas.

5. Place the pan with the quesadillas in the broiler and cook 1 to 2 minutes per side, until the tortillas are browned and crisp. Remove from the broiler and use a knife to cut each quesadilla into 4 slices. Enjoy immediately.

SIMPLE SWAP: Use shrimp in place of chicken, or omit it altogether for a vegetarian option. You can also use scrambled eggs instead of chicken for a tasty breakfast quesadilla.

PER SERVING: Calories: 349; Total fat: 15g; Saturated fat: 7g; Sodium: 520mg; Carbohydrates: 28g; Fiber: 5g; Protein: 26g; Calcium: 261mg; Potassium: 397mg

SHEET PAN CHICKEN FAJITAS

5-INGREDIENT   ONE-POT
PREP TIME: 10 minutes   **COOK TIME:** 10 minutes
SERVES 4

Give yourself an easy weeknight meal, thanks to the magic of sheet pan meals! Simply roast the chicken and veggies together, assemble the fajitas, and add your favorite toppings, such as cheese, salsa, and avocado. The chicken in this recipe can be swapped for steak, shrimp, tofu, or portobello mushrooms (cooking times may vary). This recipe can also be used as an alternate filling for Chicken and Black Bean Quesadillas (page 102).

3 cups mini sweet bell peppers or 3 bell peppers, sliced

½ red onion, sliced

1 pound boneless, skinless chicken breast, cut into thin strips

3 tablespoons avocado oil

2 tablespoons fajita seasoning

8 (6-inch) flour tortillas, warmed

1. Preheat the oven to 450°F and line a sheet pan with non-stick aluminum foil.

2. In a zip-top bag or large bowl, combine the bell peppers, onions, and chicken. Add the avocado oil and fajita seasoning. Mix to combine. Spread the mixture on the prepared sheet pan.

3. Roast the chicken and vegetables for 10 minutes, until the chicken is browned and no longer pink inside. Remove the pan from the oven, turn on the broiler to high (550°F), and place the pan under the broiler for an additional 2 minutes to brown the vegetables.

4. Fill the tortillas with the chicken-and-vegetable mixture and add your favorite toppings.

5. Save leftover chicken and vegetables in the refrigerator for up to 5 days.

COOKING HACK: Look for precut veggies for fajitas and sliced chicken strips in the meat department to cut down on prep time.

PER SERVING: Calories: 439; Total fat: 16g; Saturated fat: 3g; Sodium: 795mg; Carbohydrates: 40g; Fiber: 4g; Protein: 31g; Calcium: 98mg; Potassium: 625mg

CHICKEN MARSALA

ONE-POT

PREP TIME: 5 minutes **COOK TIME:** 25 minutes

SERVES 4

This recipe always reminds me of the holidays, with its savory and comforting mushroom-based sauce. It comes together easily and is perfect for family gatherings. Chicken tenderloins are used in place of whole breasts to provide smaller portions for more people to enjoy.

¼ cup all-purpose flour, plus 1 tablespoon

¼ teaspoon salt

¼ teaspoon freshly ground black pepper

1½ pounds chicken tenderloins

3 tablespoons olive oil, divided

1 (8-ounce) package sliced cremini mushrooms

⅔ cup marsala wine

⅔ cup low-sodium chicken broth

2 tablespoons unsalted butter

1 tablespoon fresh thyme

1. In a large zip-top bag, combine ¼ cup of flour with the salt and pepper. Add the chicken, seal the bag, and toss to coat the chicken in the flour mixture.

2. In a large skillet over medium-high heat, heat 2 tablespoons of olive oil and brown the chicken, 4 minutes per side. Work in batches, if needed. Remove the chicken from the pan and set aside.

3. Heat the remaining 1 tablespoon of oil in the skillet and sauté the mushrooms until tender, 3 minutes. Add the remaining 1 tablespoon of flour over the mushrooms, and stir constantly for 1 minute. Add the marsala wine to deglaze the pan, using a rubber spatula to scrape up any browned bits. Add the chicken broth and bring to a boil for 2 to 3 minutes, until the mixture thickens and reduces slightly.

4. Remove the pan from the heat and stir in the butter. Return the chicken to the pan and coat with the sauce. Sprinkle with the fresh thyme.

5. Store leftovers in the refrigerator for up to 5 days.

SERVING SUGGESTION: Serve this dish over pasta or zoodles, or plate with Low-Calorie Mashed Potatoes (page 134) and vegetables.

PER SERVING: Calories: 463; Total fat: 21g; Saturated fat: 6g; Sodium: 242mg; Carbohydrates: 15g; Fiber: 1g; Protein: 42g; Calcium: 21mg; Potassium: 835mg

CHICKEN WITH ROASTED RED PEPPERS, TOMATO, SPINACH, AND MELTED MOZZARELLA

PREP TIME: 5 minutes   **COOK TIME:** 10 minutes
SERVES 4

This simple weeknight meal was inspired by my local Italian eateries. The melted mozzarella cheese on top provides a comfort food feel among all the healthy, colorful vegetables. Serve with a side of whole grains, such as farro.

1½ pounds thin sliced boneless, skinless chicken breasts

2 tablespoons olive oil

2 teaspoons dried oregano, plus more for sprinkling if desired

¼ teaspoon salt

¼ teaspoon freshly ground black pepper

Nonstick cooking spray

4 cups baby spinach

½ cup jarred whole roasted red peppers, cut in half (approximately 2 whole peppers)

1 medium tomato, cut into ¼-inch-thick slices

1 (8-ounce) ball fresh mozzarella, cut into ¼-inch-thick slices

1. Preheat the oven broiler on high (550°F) and line a sheet pan with nonstick aluminum foil.

2. Season the chicken with the olive oil, oregano, salt, and pepper. Place the chicken on the prepared sheet pan and broil for 3 to 4 minutes per side until browned.

3. Heat a 10-inch nonstick skillet over medium heat and spray with cooking spray. Add the spinach and sauté until it just starts to wilt, 2 to 3 minutes. Remove the pan from the heat and set aside.

4. Remove the chicken from the broiler, keeping the broiler on. Top the chicken evenly with the roasted red peppers, tomato slices, spinach, and mozzarella. Sprinkle additional oregano on top if desired.

5. Return the pan to the broiler and heat for 2 to 3 minutes, until the cheese is melted and lightly browned on top.

6. Store any leftovers in the refrigerator for up to 3 days.

COOKING HACK: Skip the step of sautéing the spinach by using 2 cups thawed frozen spinach.

PER SERVING: Calories: 452; Total fat: 24g; Saturated fat: 9g; Sodium: 603mg; Carbohydrates: 5g; Fiber: 2g; Protein: 52g; Calcium: 337mg; Potassium: 882mg

PISTACHIO-CRUSTED CHICKEN SHEET PAN MEAL

ONE-POT

PREP TIME: 5 minutes   **COOK TIME:** 25 minutes

SERVES 4

If you're looking for an easy weeknight dinner, there's nothing better than putting everything on a pan, placing it in the oven, walking away, and coming back to a complete meal. Even the cleanup is easy when you line the sheet pan with nonstick aluminum foil. This dish features chicken with a crunch, served with herbed potatoes and veggies.

1 pound baby potatoes, halved or quartered

1 (12-ounce) package green beans

4 tablespoons olive oil, divided

1 teaspoon dried rosemary

½ teaspoon salt

½ teaspoon freshly ground black pepper

½ cup shelled pistachios, crushed

¼ cup panko bread crumbs

2 tablespoons Dijon mustard

1 pound thin sliced boneless, skinless chicken breasts

1. Preheat the oven to 475°F. Line a sheet pan with non-stick foil.

2. In a large zip-top bag or bowl, toss the potatoes and green beans with 2 tablespoons of olive oil, rosemary, salt, and pepper to coat. Spread the vegetables on the prepared sheet pan and roast for 10 minutes.

3. In a medium shallow bowl, mix together the crushed pistachios and panko bread crumbs.

4. In a small bowl, whisk together the remaining 2 tablespoons of olive oil with the Dijon. Use a brush to coat the chicken with the Dijon-oil mixture, then cover it on both sides with the panko-pistachio mix.

5. Remove the pan with the vegetables from the oven. Toss the potatoes and green beans, then push them aside to create a space in the middle of the pan for the chicken. Place the chicken on the pan and bake for an additional 15 to 18 minutes, until the topping is browned and the chicken is cooked through (internal temperature of 165°F).

6. Store leftovers in the refrigerator for up to 3 days.

COOKING HACK: The smaller the potatoes, the faster they will cook. Look for bags of small baby potatoes in your produce section.

PER SERVING: Calories: 508; Total fat: 24g; Saturated fat: 3g; Sodium: 557mg; Carbohydrates: 42g; Fiber: 7g; Protein: 34g; Calcium: 112mg; Potassium: 1,142mg

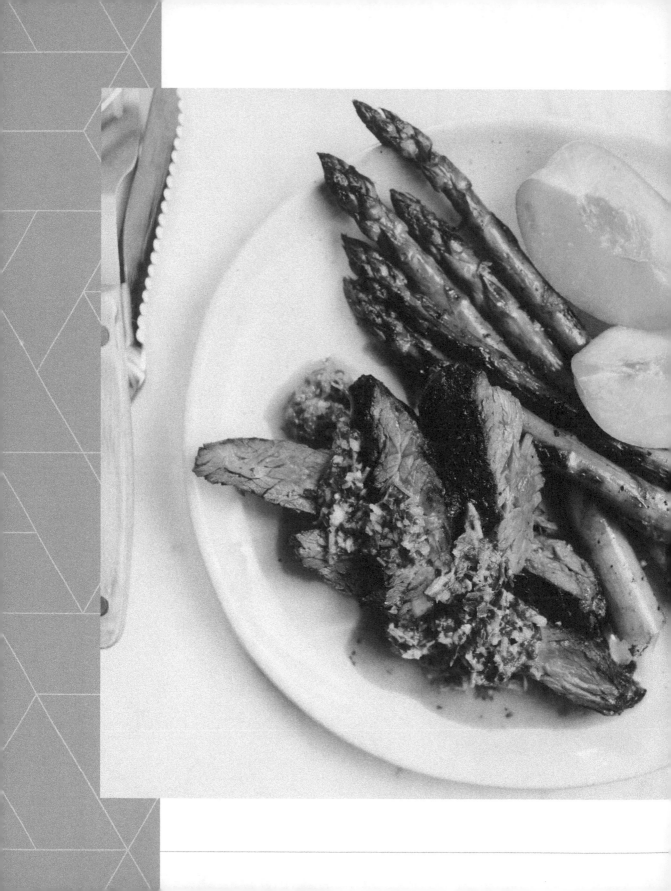

Beef, Pork, and Lamb

To lose weight or be healthy, many people think you need to avoid proteins like beef, pork, and lamb. However, all healthy eating lifestyle recommendations incorporate these meats to some degree. You can enjoy meat a few times a week in moderation. Keep in mind that meat doesn't have to be the primary component of a meal; it can be a supporting cast member in meals starring vegetables or grains.

SWEET CHILI BEEF AND VEGETABLE STIR-FRY

5-INGREDIENT   EXTRA LOW CALORIE   ONE-POT
PREP TIME: 5 minutes   **COOK TIME:** 15 minutes
SERVES 4

I always keep a variety of sauces on hand to put together quick meals. This stir-fry works great with any sauce. I love the flavor of sweet chili sauce, but it can be high in added sugars, so look for options sweetened with fruit juice instead of sugar, such as Yai's Thai. Enjoy this stir-fry with rice, or for a low-carb option, try it with shirataki or kohlrabi noodles.

2 tablespoons avocado oil, divided

1 pound lean beef, such as sirloin or flank, cut into strips

1 (12-ounce) bag fresh broccoli florets, chopped small

1 red bell pepper, cut into thin strips

1 (8-ounce) container sliced mushrooms

½ cup sweet chili sauce

1. In a large nonstick skillet or wok, heat 1 tablespoon of oil over medium heat. Add the beef and cook, stirring frequently, until no longer pink, 5 minutes. Remove the beef from the pan.

2. In the same skillet, heat the remaining 1 tablespoon of oil. Add the broccoli and stir-fry for 1 minute.

3. Add the peppers and mushrooms and cook, stirring frequently, until the vegetables are just tender and the broccoli is bright green, 4 to 5 minutes.

4. Return the beef to the pan and stir to combine. Add the sweet chili sauce, reduce the heat to medium-low, and stir to coat the meat and vegetables until the sauce is heated through and thickened, 1 to 2 minutes. Serve immediately.

5. Store leftovers in a sealed container in the refrigerator for 3 to 4 days.

COOKING HACK: Look for precut stir-fry strips in the butcher department and prepped stir-fry vegetables in the produce department.

PER SERVING: Calories: 303; Total fat: 13g; Saturated fat: 3g; Sodium: 549mg; Carbohydrates: 16g; Fiber: 5g; Protein: 30g; Calcium: 74mg; Potassium: 1,045mg

BEEF AND ZUCCHINI SKILLET LASAGNA

EXTRA LOW CALORIE   ONE-POT

PREP TIME: 5 minutes   **COOK TIME:** 15 minutes

SERVES 6

Lasagna gets a healthier makeover with this express one-pan version. This recipe swaps lasagna noodles with zucchini noodles—aka "zoodles"—for a low-carb option that cooks in less time than it takes to assemble a traditional lasagna. Even the most die-hard lasagna lover will enjoy this skillet, especially when they see how quickly dinner reaches the table.

1 pound lean ground beef

Salt

Freshly ground black pepper

2 garlic cloves, minced

1 (24-ounce) jar marinara sauce (I recommend Rao's)

1½ pounds prepared zucchini noodles (from 2 medium zucchini)

½ cup shredded part-skim mozzarella cheese

4 tablespoons shredded Parmesan cheese

¾ cup part-skim ricotta cheese

¼ cup fresh basil, chopped

1. Put the beef in a large nonstick skillet over medium-high heat, season with salt and pepper, and sauté until browned, 5 minutes.

2. Add the garlic and sauté for another minute. Pour in the marinara sauce and stir to combine.

3. Place the zoodles on top, cover, and cook for 2 to 3 minutes, until the zoodles are softened but still crisp.

4. Remove the pan from the heat. Add ¼ cup of mozzarella and 2 tablespoons of Parmesan cheese. Stir to combine with the zoodles and beef. Place dollops of ricotta around the top, sprinkle on the remaining ¼ cup of mozzarella and 2 tablespoons of Parmesan, cover, and let sit for 3 to 5 minutes, until the cheese is melted. Top with the basil and serve immediately.

5. Store any leftovers in a sealed container in the refrigerator for 3 to 5 days.

COOKING HACK: Buy premade zoodles in the produce department to cut down on prep time or if you don't own a spiralizer—one less thing to clean!

PER SERVING: Calories: 272; Total fat: 14g; Saturated fat: 6g; Sodium: 257mg; Carbohydrates: 13g; Fiber: 3g; Protein: 27g; Calcium: 247mg; Potassium: 1,188mg

FLANK STEAK WITH CHIMICHURRI SAUCE

ONE-POT

PREP TIME: 5 minutes   **COOK TIME:** 15 minutes

SERVES 4

Chimichurri is a zesty Argentinian version of pesto sauce that doubles as a marinade. It provides a ton of fresh flavor to meat, seafood, chicken, and even vegetables. Serve this dish alongside asparagus and Low-Calorie Mashed Potatoes (page 134) or Quinoa with Toasted Pine Nuts and Tomato (page 133).

¾ cup flat-leaf parsley, packed

¼ cup cilantro, packed

2 tablespoons fresh oregano

1 small shallot, quartered

3 garlic cloves

½ teaspoon kosher salt, plus more for seasoning

½ teaspoon freshly ground black pepper, plus more for seasoning

1 tablespoon lemon juice

¼ cup red wine vinegar

¼ teaspoon red pepper flakes

¾ cup extra-virgin olive oil

1½ pounds flank steak

1. Preheat a grill or grill pan over medium-high heat.

2. In a food processor or blender, combine the parsley, cilantro, oregano, shallot, garlic, salt, pepper, and lemon juice. Pulse to combine, scraping down the sides with a rubber spatula. Add the vinegar and red pepper flakes and pulse again to blend. Drizzle with the olive oil while pulsing to blend.

3. Season the steak with salt, pepper, and 1 tablespoon of chimichurri sauce per side. Grill for 5 to 6 minutes per side, then remove from the heat and tent with aluminum foil for 5 minutes before slicing. Serve with chimichurri sauce drizzled on top.

4. Store the steak and sauce separately in the refrigerator for up to 4 days.

LOVE YOUR LEFTOVERS: Make a breakfast steak and eggs with leftover steak and sauce, or enjoy a steak salad for lunch.

PER SERVING: Calories: 485; Total fat: 35g; Saturated fat: 7g; Sodium: 245mg; Carbohydrates: 2g; Fiber: 1g; Protein: 37g; Calcium: 58mg; Potassium: 675mg

FILET MIGNON WITH BLACK PEPPERCORN–MUSHROOM SAUCE

PREP TIME: 5 minutes   **COOK TIME:** 25 minutes
SERVES 4

If you're looking for an easy-but-fancy dinner, this is the recipe for you. The savory, umami sauce is a perfect complement to the tender steak. Serve with Cauliflower Risotto (page 130), Low-Calorie Mashed Potatoes (page 134), or Rosemary-Parmesan Smashed Potatoes (page 135) to soak up the sauce.

4 (5-ounce) filet mignon steaks, 2 inches thick

Salt

Freshly ground black pepper

2 tablespoons unsalted butter

1 (8-ounce) container sliced cremini or white mushrooms

⅓ cup minced shallots

1 garlic clove, minced

½ cup red wine

1½ cups beef broth

1 tablespoon whole peppercorns, coarsely crushed

2 tablespoons water

1 tablespoon cornstarch

1. Preheat a grill or grill pan over high heat.

2. Season the steaks with salt and pepper and set aside.

3. Heat a medium heavy-bottomed saucepan over medium heat. Melt the butter, then sauté the mushrooms and shallots until softened, 5 minutes. Add the garlic and sauté for 30 seconds until fragrant. Stir in the wine to deglaze the pan, using a spatula to scrape up any browned bits, then add the broth and peppercorns.

4. In a small bowl, whisk together the water and cornstarch. Stir the cornstarch mixture into the sauce. Simmer over medium heat, stirring frequently, until the liquid is reduced and thickened, 10 to 15 minutes. Reduce the heat to low to keep the sauce warm.

5. If cooking on the grill, sear the steaks over high direct heat for 3 minutes per side, then transfer to indirect heat for 9 minutes. This will result in a medium-cooked steak (internal temperature of 145°F). If using a grill pan or cast-iron pan, sear the steaks over high heat for 3 minutes per side, then transfer the pan to a 425°F oven for 9 minutes. Transfer the steaks to a plate and tent with aluminum foil for 5 minutes. Serve with the sauce.

6. Store leftover steak and sauce separately in the refrigerator for 3 to 5 days. Reheat the sauce on the stovetop, adding additional broth to thin the sauce if needed.

PER SERVING: Calories: 470; Total fat: 32g; Saturated fat: 14g; Sodium: 462mg; Carbohydrates: 9g; Fiber: 2g; Protein: 30g; Calcium: 54mg; Potassium: 698mg

THREE-MEAT AND MUSHROOM MEATBALLS

EXTRA LOW CALORIE

PREP TIME: 10 minutes   **COOK TIME:** 25 minutes
SERVES 6

These meatballs illustrate how you can stretch your meat by adding mushrooms. Using a blend of meat and mushrooms helps cut down on saturated fat while increasing moistness and adding a savory umami flavor. Enjoy these yummy meatballs on their own, over pasta, or with Spicy Garlicky Zoodles (page 129) for a kick. A blend of beef, pork, and veal provides a juicier flavor, but feel free to use all beef instead.

1 (8-ounce) package sliced mushrooms

1 pound ground beef, veal, and pork mix

2 tablespoons Italian seasoning

2 tablespoons grated Parmesan cheese

2 tablespoons seasoned bread crumbs

1 large egg

1 garlic clove, minced

1. Preheat the oven to 400°F and line a sheet pan with non-stick aluminum foil.

2. Pulse the mushrooms in a food processor to finely chop.

3. Preheat a small nonstick skillet over medium heat, add the mushrooms, and sauté until they're browned and have released their liquid, 3 minutes. Drain the liquid and transfer the mushrooms to a large bowl.

4. To the same bowl, add the ground meat, Italian seasoning, Parmesan, bread crumbs, egg, and garlic. Use your hands to mix everything until combined, then roll into 1½-inch balls and place them on the prepared sheet pan, 1 inch apart.

5. Bake for 20 minutes, until cooked through (internal temperature of 160°F). Transfer the meatballs to a plate lined with a paper towel to absorb any excess fat.

6. Store leftover meatballs in the refrigerator for 3 to 5 days, or freeze for 3 to 4 months.

COOKING HACK: Place the meatballs on a baking rack on the sheet pan to catch drippings. This will result in firmer meatballs and drain off excess fat.

PER SERVING: Calories: 161; Total fat: 9g; Saturated fat: 3g; Sodium: 134mg; Carbohydrates: 2g; Fiber: 0g; Protein: 18g; Calcium: 30mg; Potassium: 379mg

TERIYAKI PORK AND PINEAPPLE STIR-FRY

5-INGREDIENT   EXTRA LOW CALORIE   ONE-POT
PREP TIME: 5 minutes   **COOK TIME:** 15 minutes
SERVES 4

Stir-fries are fantastic weeknight meals, because they come together fast and are a great way to use up vegetables. Serve this tasty stir-fry with rice or noodles and garnish with sesame seeds, if desired. Look for a low-sodium teriyaki sauce option, such as Kikkoman.

2 tablespoons avocado
   oil, divided

2 red bell peppers, sliced

1 cup snow peas

Salt

Freshly ground black pepper

1 pound boneless pork chops,
   cut into 1-inch cubes

1 cup pineapple chunks

½ cup teriyaki sauce

1. In a large nonstick skillet or wok, heat 1 tablespoon of oil over medium-high heat. Add the peppers and snow peas and season with salt and pepper. Cook for 3 minutes, stirring frequently, until the peppers are slightly tender. Remove the peppers and snow peas from the pan and set aside.

2. In the same skillet, heat the remaining 1 tablespoon of oil. Add the pork, season with salt and pepper, and cook for 5 minutes, stirring frequently, until the pork is browned and cooked through.

3. Add the pineapple and toss with the meat for 1 minute. Return the peppers and snow peas to the skillet and stir to combine. Add the teriyaki sauce and toss to coat. Cook for an additional 2 to 3 minutes, until the sauce comes to a boil and thickens slightly. Remove from the heat and serve immediately.

4. Store leftover stir-fry in the refrigerator for up to 4 days.

COOKING HACK: Look for precut pineapple in the produce department or used canned pineapple chunks with the juices drained. If you use canned pineapples, make sure the pineapple is canned in its own juices.

PER SERVING: Calories: 316; Total fat: 11g; Saturated fat: 2g; Sodium: 739mg; Carbohydrates: 24g; Fiber: 2g; Protein: 29g; Calcium: 31mg; Potassium: 738mg

PORK MILANESE

PREP TIME: 10 minutes   **COOK TIME:** 10 minutes
SERVES 4

"Milanese style" calls for thin slices of meat dredged in eggs and seasoned bread crumbs and then lightly fried. It looks really fancy but comes together in no time. This is topped with an arugula salad mixture to optimize nutrition. Try this recipe with chicken or seafood fillets as well.

4 boneless pork chops

½ cup all-purpose flour

2 large eggs, beaten

1 cup seasoned bread crumbs

6 tablespoons olive oil, divided

4 cups arugula

Juice of 1 lemon

Salt

Freshly ground black pepper

½ cup grape tomatoes, halved

¼ cup shaved Parmesan cheese

1. Place a pork chop between two pieces of plastic wrap. Using a mallet, pound the pork chop thin. Repeat with the remaining chops.

2. Place the flour, eggs, and bread crumbs in individual shallow dishes. Dip the pork in the flour to coat, then dip into the egg, and then into the bread crumbs.

3. In a large nonstick skillet, heat 2 tablespoons of oil over medium heat.

4. Place the breaded pork into the skillet. Cooking in batches if needed, cook for 4 minutes per side, or until browned and crisp. Transfer the cutlets to a plate lined with paper towels to absorb excess oil.

5. In a medium bowl, toss the arugula together with the lemon juice and remaining 4 tablespoons of oil, and season with salt and pepper. Stir in the tomatoes.

6. Place the pork on individual plates, top with the arugula mixture, and sprinkle with the Parmesan.

7. Store any leftover pork without the arugula mixture in the refrigerator for up to 4 days. Save the greens separately or make a fresh batch when serving.

COOKING HACK: Your butcher department may be able to pound the pork chops for you at the store.

PER SERVING: Calories: 516; Total fat: 30g; Saturated fat: 6g; Sodium: 313mg; Carbohydrates: 20g; Fiber: 1g; Protein: 39g; Calcium: 124mg; Potassium: 755mg

PORK AND KIMCHI FRIED RICE

PREP TIME: 5 minutes   **COOK TIME:** 20 minutes
SERVES 4

Give your fried rice some heat by adding kimchi. Made from fermented vegetables, kimchi is an excellent source of probiotics for gut health. A healthy gut may also play a role in our metabolism. Enjoy this as a meal or serve as a side dish.

3 tablespoons canola oil, divided

2 large eggs, beaten

1 cup diced yellow onions

3 scallions, thinly sliced

1 garlic clove, minced

1 pound ground pork

Salt

Freshly ground black pepper

1 cup frozen peas and carrots

1 (9-ounce) package precooked brown rice

1 cup chopped kimchi

3 tablespoons gochujang paste (optional)

1. In a large nonstick skillet, heat 1 tablespoon of oil over high heat. Add the eggs and cook without stirring for 30 seconds, until the eggs are set. Flip and cook for another 15 to 30 seconds. Remove the eggs from the pan and cut into ½-inch pieces. Set aside.

2. In the same skillet, heat another 1 tablespoon of oil and add the onions. Sauté until the onions are translucent, 2 to 3 minutes.

3. Add the scallions and garlic and sauté for another 30 seconds, until softened.

4. Add the pork, season with salt and pepper, and sauté while breaking up the meat until cooked through and no longer pink, 5 minutes.

5. Add the frozen peas and carrots and stir together with the pork until heated through, 1 to 2 minutes. Transfer the pork and vegetables to a medium bowl.

6. In the same skillet, heat the remaining 1 tablespoon of oil. Add the precooked rice, spread thin to cover the bottom of the pan, and let it sit in the pan for a minute to brown. Stir for 5 minutes, occasionally spreading the rice into a flat layer in the pan to crisp. Return the pork, vegetables, and eggs back to the skillet, add the kimchi and gochujang (if using), and stir until combined. Serve immediately.

7. Store leftovers in the refrigerator for 5 to 7 days.

COOKING HACK: Day-old rice or precooked rice available in microwave packets is drier and will cook best for fried rice.

PER SERVING: Calories: 544; Total fat: 38g; Saturated fat: 11g; Sodium: 236mg; Carbohydrates: 25g; Fiber: 4g; Protein: 27g; Calcium: 88mg; Potassium: 634mg

COFFEE-RUBBED PORK FOIL PACKETS WITH MANGO SALSA

EXTRA LOW CALORIE   ONE-POT
PREP TIME: 10 minutes   **COOK TIME:** 20 minutes
SERVES 4

Did you know coffee makes an amazing rub for meats? The acidity of coffee tenderizes the meat while sealing in flavor. Cooking the meat in foil packets creates a super juicy chop. Premade coffee rubs can be found in the spice section of the grocery store, or make your own using 1 tablespoon each of ground coffee, brown sugar, onion powder, and paprika with 1 teaspoon each of black pepper, salt, and chili powder.

2 tablespoons coffee rub

1 pound boneless pork chops, ½ inch thick

1 orange, cut into ¼-inch-thick slices

1 red onion, half sliced and half diced

2 cups diced mango

1 jalapeño, seeded and minced (optional)

¼ cup chopped fresh cilantro

Juice of 1 lime

1. Preheat the oven to 450ºF. Tear off 4 pieces of aluminum foil, 14 inches in length.

2. Using your hands, massage the coffee rub into both sides of the pork chops and place a chop in the middle of each piece of foil. Lay the orange slices and onion slices on top of the pork.

3. Bring the long ends of the foil together, fold down to seal in the pork, then fold in the sides on top to create packets. Place the packets directly on the middle oven rack and bake for 16 to 18 minutes, until the pork is cooked through (internal temperature of 160ºF).

4. In a small bowl, combine the mango, diced onion, jalapeño (if using), cilantro, and lime juice.

5. Remove the foil packets from the oven and open them carefully to avoid the steam. Discard the orange and onion slices and transfer the pork chops onto plates. Top the pork with the mango salsa.

6. Store leftover chops in the refrigerator for 3 to 4 days. Stored separately, the mango salsa will keep in the refrigerator for up to 5 days.

PER SERVING: Calories: 222; Total fat: 4g; Saturated fat: 1g; Sodium: 123mg; Carbohydrates: 20g; Fiber: 3g; Protein: 27g; Calcium: 36mg; Potassium: 688mg

MAPLE-MUSTARD SHEET PAN PORK CHOPS WITH BRUSSELS SPROUTS

5-INGREDIENT   EXTRA LOW CALORIE   ONE-POT
PREP TIME: 5 minutes   **COOK TIME:** 25 minutes
SERVES 4

Maple syrup and mustard make a sweet-savory combination that pairs perfectly with pork and roasted veggies. Use pure maple syrup, a natural sweetener. A little goes a long way and provides caramelization while roasting.

1 pound Brussels sprouts, trimmed and halved or quartered

3 tablespoons olive oil, divided

3 tablespoons maple syrup, divided

2 tablespoons apple cider vinegar, divided

Salt

Freshly ground black pepper

¼ cup whole-grain mustard

1 pound boneless pork chops, ½ inch thick

1. Preheat the oven to 450°F. Line a sheet pan with nonstick aluminum foil.

2. In a medium bowl or zip-top bag, toss the Brussels sprouts with 2 tablespoons of olive oil, 1 tablespoon of maple syrup, and 1 tablespoon of vinegar.

3. Spread the Brussels sprouts on the sheet pan, season with salt and pepper, and roast for 10 to 15 minutes, until they just start to brown.

4. In the same medium bowl, whisk together the remaining 1 tablespoon of olive oil, remaining 2 tablespoons of maple syrup, remaining 1 tablespoon of vinegar, and the mustard. Toss with the pork chops to marinate.

5. Remove the sheet pan from the oven. Flip the Brussels sprouts and move them aside so they fill two-thirds of the pan. Line the pork chops along one short edge of the pan. Roast for an additional 10 minutes, until the pork is cooked through (internal temperature of 160°F).

6. Store any leftovers in the refrigerator for up to 5 days.

COOKING HACK: Cut cook time by using shaved Brussels sprouts and roasting the pork and sprouts together for 10 to 15 minutes.

PER SERVING: Calories: 323; Total fat: 14g; Saturated fat: 3g; Sodium: 125mg; Carbohydrates: 20g; Fiber: 4g; Protein: 29g; Calcium: 69mg; Potassium: 917mg

LAMB TACOS WITH CUCUMBER, TOMATO, AND GOAT CHEESE

ONE-POT

PREP TIME: 10 minutes **COOK TIME:** 10 minutes

SERVES 4

Two great street foods come together in this recipe: tacos and gyros. These Mediterranean-style tacos are a lightened-up version of a traditional gyro, which can often cost you 600 to 700 in calories. In addition to a cucumber-tomato mixture and goat cheese, top off your tacos with Kalamata olives, chopped romaine, fresh mint, or parsley.

½ seedless English cucumber, small diced

1 cup grape tomatoes, quartered

Salt

Freshly ground black pepper

1 tablespoon olive oil

3 garlic cloves, minced

1 pound ground lamb

2 tablespoons Greek seasoning blend

2 tablespoons tomato paste

8 (6-inch) whole-wheat flour tortillas, warmed

¼ cup goat cheese crumbles

½ cup Tzatziki Sauce (page 141) or store-bought sauce

1. In a small bowl, combine the cucumber and tomatoes. Season with salt and pepper and set aside.

2. In a large nonstick skillet, heat the oil over medium heat. Add the garlic and cook until fragrant, 30 seconds.

3. Add the ground lamb and Greek seasoning. Use a wooden spoon to break up the meat and combine it with the garlic and seasonings. Cook for 5 minutes, or until browned and cooked through.

4. Add the tomato paste and stir until combined, 1 to 2 minutes. Remove from heat.

5. Assemble the tacos on tortillas with the lamb, cucumber-tomato mixture, goat cheese crumbles, and tzatziki sauce.

6. Store leftover lamb mixture in the refrigerator for up to 5 days.

SERVING SUGGESTION: Serve these tacos with a Greek salad, such as the base of the Falafel Bowl (page 51), or use the lamb taco meat in place of the falafel in the Falafel Bowl for a low-carb bowl.

PER SERVING: Calories: 516; Total fat: 23g; Saturated fat: 8g; Sodium: 454mg; Carbohydrates: 39g; Fiber: 7g; Protein: 32g; Calcium: 149mg; Potassium: 732mg

SPINACH AND FETA LAMB BURGERS

5-INGREDIENT   EXTRA LOW CALORIE   ONE-POT
PREP TIME: 5 minutes   **COOK TIME:** 10 minutes
SERVES 4

This juicy and savory burger with a Mediterranean flair calls for lamb, salty feta cheese, and fresh spinach—a fun change-up to the usual backyard barbecue or tailgate. Serve as regular-size burgers or create smaller patties for sliders. Enjoy them on a bun, in pita bread, or on a salad. You can also use them in place of the falafel in the Falafel Bowl (page 51).

1 pound ground lamb

1 tablespoon Greek seasoning blend

½ cup crumbled feta cheese

1 cup chopped baby spinach

Tzatziki Sauce (page 141) or store-bought sauce, for topping

1. Preheat a grill or grill pan over medium-high heat.

2. In a large bowl, combine the lamb, Greek seasoning, feta, and spinach. Using your hands, incorporate the ingredients and shape into 4 patties.

3. Grill the burgers for 4 minutes per side for a medium-cooked burger (internal temperature of 145°F). Serve immediately with tzatziki sauce drizzled on top.

4. Store cooked burgers in the refrigerator for 3 to 4 days. Alternatively, you can freeze raw burgers individually wrapped and stored in a freezer-safe bag for 3 to 4 months.

SERVING SUGGESTION: Top the burgers with a slice of roasted red pepper and romaine lettuce.

PER SERVING: Calories: 279; Total fat: 19g; Saturated fat: 9g; Sodium: 250mg; Carbohydrates: 2g; Fiber: 0g; Protein: 26g; Calcium: 123mg; Potassium: 396mg

ZA'ATAR LAMB KEBABS WITH HERBED YOGURT SAUCE

EXTRA LOW CALORIE   ONE-POT
PREP TIME: 15 minutes   **COOK TIME:** 10 minutes
SERVES 4

Za'atar is a Middle Eastern herb that's often blended with sesame seeds, sumac, and salt into a spice mixture called za'atar blend. You can create your own za'atar blend, but when it's readily available for purchase, why not skip that step and get going on your meal?

1 pound boneless lamb meat, cut into 1-inch cubes

Zest and juice of 1 lemon, divided

1 tablespoon olive oil, plus ¼ cup

3 tablespoons za'atar seasoning blend, divided

½ cup plain nonfat Greek yogurt

1 tablespoon chopped fresh mint

1 tablespoon chopped fresh parsley

Freshly ground black pepper

1 red onion, halved, then quartered

8 mini bell peppers, halved

8 ounces whole mushrooms

1. Preheat a grill or grill pan over medium-high heat.

2. In a zip-top bag or medium bowl, combine the lamb, juice from half a lemon, 1 tablespoon of oil, and 1 tablespoon of za'atar seasoning together to coat the meat.

3. In a small bowl, whisk together the remaining ¼ cup of olive oil and remaining 2 tablespoons of za'atar seasoning. Set aside.

4. In a separate small bowl, whisk together the yogurt, mint, parsley, the remaining lemon juice, lemon zest, and pepper to taste. Refrigerate the sauce until the lamb is ready.

5. Assemble the skewers by alternating the onion, peppers, mushrooms, and lamb. Brush the vegetables with the oil-and-za'atar mixture. Grill the skewers over medium-high heat for 8 minutes, turning skewers a quarter turn every 2 minutes. Serve immediately with the chilled sauce.

6. To store leftovers, remove the meat and veggies from the skewers and store in the refrigerator for up to 2 days.

TECHNIQUE TRICK: If using wooden skewers, soak them for at least 15 minutes before assembling to prevent them from catching fire on the grill.

PER SERVING: Calories: 305; Total fat: 17g; Saturated fat: 4g; Sodium: 108mg; Carbohydrates: 10g; Fiber: 2g; Protein: 28g; Calcium: 57mg; Potassium: 742mg

LAMB BOLOGNESE WITH PAPPARDELLE

PREP TIME: 5 minutes   **COOK TIME:** 25 minutes

SERVES 4

Marinara is my go-to sauce, but when I want to kick things up, I upgrade to a Bolognese. This hearty sauce typically simmers for hours to become thick and flavorful, but my express version uses store-bought marinara sauce (I recommend Rao's), in which the flavors have already come together, along with ground lamb meat for a stronger flavor than beef.

1 tablespoon olive oil

½ yellow onion, diced

1 celery stalk, diced

1 carrot, peeled and diced

1 garlic clove, minced

1 pound ground lamb

½ cup red wine

1 (24-ounce) jar marinara sauce

1 pound pappardelle pasta, cooked per package instructions

Shredded Parmesan cheese, for garnish (optional)

Chopped basil, for garnish (optional)

1. In a large stockpot, heat the oil over medium-high heat.

2. Add the onion, celery, and carrot and sauté until the onion is translucent and the vegetables are tender, 5 minutes.

3. Add the garlic and sauté for 30 seconds, until fragrant. Add the lamb and cook, breaking apart with a spoon, until no longer pink, 3 minutes.

4. Add the wine to deglaze the pot, using the spoon to scrape up any browned bits, then stir in the marinara sauce. Bring the sauce to a boil, then cover and simmer over medium-low heat for 15 minutes. Serve immediately with pasta and garnish with Parmesan cheese and chopped basil (if using).

5. Store the sauce and pasta separately in the refrigerator for up to 5 days or freeze for 3 months.

SIMPLE SWAP: A wide pasta noodle works best with Bolognese, so if you'd like, swap the pappardelle for tagliatelle or fettucine. Alternatively, farro offers a high-fiber whole-grain option, while zoodles are a nice low-carb option.

PER SERVING: Calories: 750; Total fat: 20g; Saturated fat: 6g; Sodium: 105mg; Carbohydrates: 98g; Fiber: 7g; Protein: 40g; Calcium: 63mg; Potassium: 1,160mg

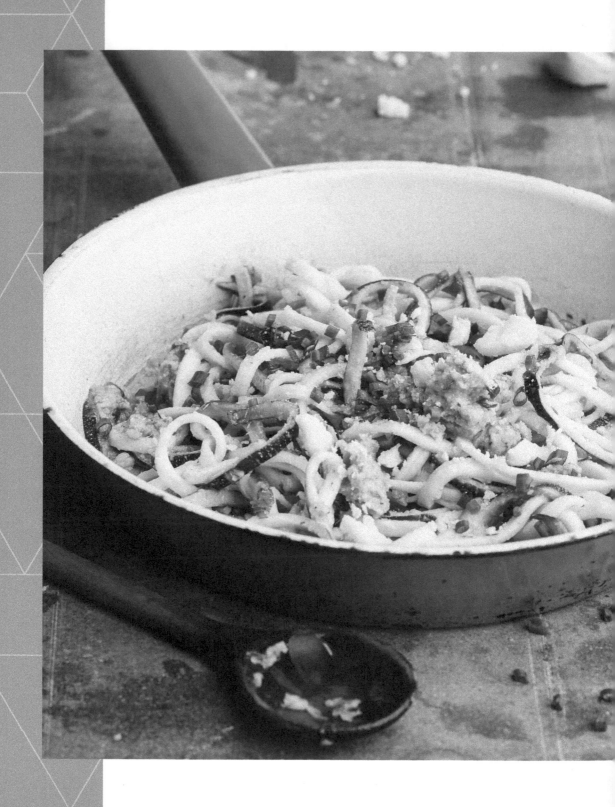

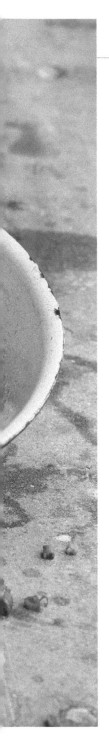

CHAPTER EIGHT

Sides, Dressings, and Sauces

For a complete meal, you'll want to round out your plate with side dishes that can add extra fiber and protein. The following pages offer suggestions for pairings with many of the recipes in this book. A side shouldn't compete with a main dish for flavor; rather, it should enhance the meal. You'll also find dressings and sauces that can add a boost of flavor to dishes. Store-bought versions are convenient, but making your own gives you control over the ingredients and calories. Now, turn the page and let's finish off those meals!

SPICY GARLICKY ZOODLES

5-INGREDIENT   EXTRA LOW CALORIE   ONE-POT
PREP TIME: 5 minutes   **COOK TIME:** 5 minutes
SERVES 4

I'm a big fan of convenience cuts at the grocery store, and that especially holds true for spiralized vegetables, readily available in most produce departments. Zucchini noodles (better known as zoodles) are not just a low-carb alternative to pasta—they're also a fun way to enjoy vegetables. Pre-spiralized zucchini makes this quick side dish plate-ready in under 10 minutes.

1 tablespoon olive oil

4 garlic cloves, minced

1 teaspoon red pepper flakes

1 pound zucchini, spiralized

¼ teaspoon salt

Grated Parmesan cheese, for garnish (optional)

1. In a large nonstick skillet, heat the oil over medium heat. Add the garlic and red pepper flakes and sauté until fragrant, about 30 seconds.

2. Stir in the zoodles to combine with the garlic and red pepper flakes and sauté until softened, 4 minutes.

3. Season the zoodles with salt and garnish with Parmesan cheese (if using).

4. Store leftover cooked zoodles in the refrigerator for up to 2 days.

SIMPLE SWAP: If you prefer a less spicy side dish, create lemon-herb zoodles instead. Swap the red pepper flakes for 1 teaspoon dried herbs such as basil or oregano. At the end, stir in 3 tablespoons lemon juice and sprinkle with salt and freshly ground black pepper.

PER SERVING: Calories: 54; Total fat: 4g; Saturated fat: 1g; Sodium: 155mg; Carbohydrates: 5g; Fiber: 1g; Protein: 2g; Calcium: 24mg; Potassium: 308mg

CAULIFLOWER RISOTTO

5-INGREDIENT   EXTRA LOW CALORIE   ONE-POT
PREP TIME: 5 minutes   **COOK TIME:** 15 minutes
SERVES 2

I love risotto, but I don't enjoy standing over my stove continuously stirring it for an hour when I make it at home. This cauliflower rice version cooks quickly with minimal stirring and offers a low-carb swap to an otherwise indulgent side dish. It's still got a great cheesy flavor.

2 tablespoons olive oil

2 garlic cloves, minced

1 (12-ounce) package fresh cauliflower rice (about 2 cups)

1 cup vegetable stock or broth

1 cup shredded or grated Parmesan cheese

1 teaspoon dried thyme

1. In a medium nonstick skillet, heat the oil over medium heat. Add the garlic and sauté for 1 to 2 minutes, until translucent.

2. Stir in the cauliflower to coat with the oil and add the broth. Simmer, stirring occasionally, for 10 minutes, until the liquid is absorbed.

3. Remove the skillet from the heat and stir in the Parmesan cheese and thyme. Serve immediately.

4. Store leftover risotto in the refrigerator for up to 2 days.

SERVING SUGGESTION: Serve this risotto along with a saucy dish, such as Filet Mignon with Black Peppercorn–Mushroom Sauce (page 114) or Chicken Marsala (page 104), so the cauliflower can soak up the liquid.

PER SERVING: Calories: 383; Total fat: 28g; Saturated fat: 10g; Sodium: 932mg; Carbohydrates: 18g; Fiber: 4g; Protein: 17g; Calcium: 471mg; Potassium: 613mg

ROASTED SHAVED BRUSSELS SPROUTS

5-INGREDIENT   EXTRA LOW CALORIE   ONE-POT
PREP TIME: 5 minutes   **COOK TIME:** 15 minutes
SERVES 2

Shaved Brussels sprouts roast faster and crispier than whole Brussels sprouts.
I became a fan immediately. This recipe's simple seasoning allows you to enjoy
the natural sweetness of the roasted greens, but I encourage you to experiment
with other herbs and seasonings as well, such as lemon pepper. You can also enjoy
shaved sprouts raw in salads—try swapping them for the kale in the Kale Caesar
Salad (page 41).

1 pound Brussels
  sprouts, shaved

¼ cup olive oil

½ teaspoon salt, plus more
  for seasoning

½ teaspoon freshly ground
  black pepper, plus more
  for seasoning

Parmesan cheese, for garnish
  (optional)

1. Preheat the oven to 450°F. Line a sheet pan with parchment
   paper or nonstick aluminum foil.

2. In a large bowl, toss the shaved Brussels sprouts with the
   olive oil, salt, and pepper. Spread them out into a single
   layer on the prepared sheet pan. Season with additional
   salt and pepper as needed.

3. Roast the Brussels sprouts for 15 minutes, until browned
   and crisp. Remove them from the oven and sprinkle on the
   Parmesan cheese (if using).

4. Store any leftover Brussels sprouts in the refrigerator for up
   to 3 days. Reheat in a 350°F oven for 5 minutes to re-crisp.

TECHNIQUE TRICK: If you can't find pre-shredded Brussels sprouts in
the produce department, run trimmed and peeled Brussels sprouts
through a food processor with a shredding blade.

PER SERVING: Calories: 336; Total fat: 28g; Saturated fat: 4g;
Sodium: 639mg; Carbohydrates: 20g; Fiber: 9g; Protein: 8g;
Calcium: 96mg; Potassium: 886mg

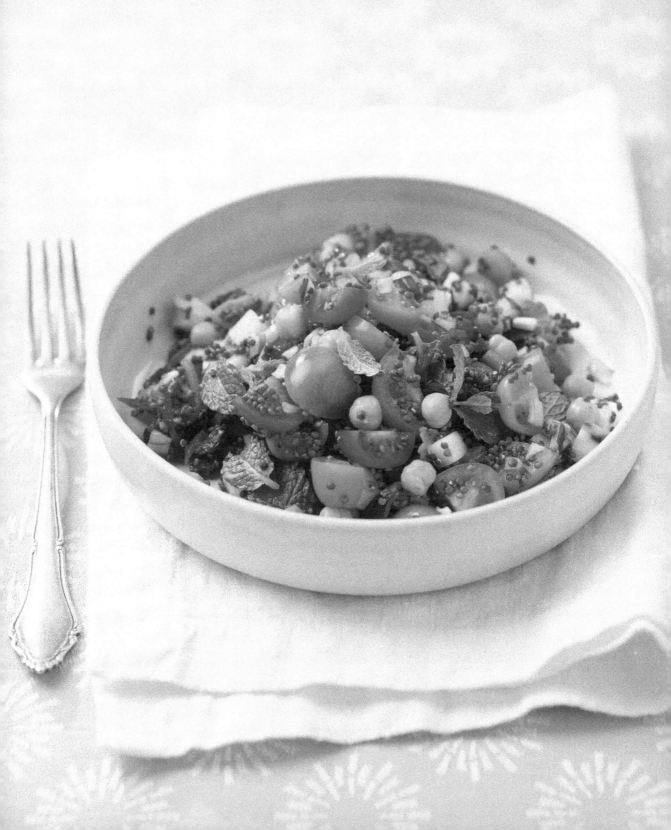

QUINOA WITH TOASTED PINE NUTS AND TOMATO

EXTRA LOW CALORIE   ONE-POT

PREP TIME: 5 minutes   **COOK TIME:** 25 minutes

SERVES 4

Create a quick pilaf using quinoa, toasted pine nuts, and sweet tomatoes. Quinoa provides fiber and protein for added satisfaction and helps with weight management. This dish makes a delicious side served along dishes like Fish en Papillote (page 97). It's also great as the base of a grain bowl, such as the Pesto Grain Bowl with Chickpeas (page 50).

¼ cup pine nuts

2 tablespoons olive oil

½ sweet onion, diced

1 cup uncooked quinoa

1½ cups low-sodium chicken broth

½ cup halved grape tomatoes

¼ cup chopped fresh parsley

Juice of ½ lemon

1. In an ungreased medium saucepan over medium heat, toast the pine nuts by continuously tossing them until fragrant and browned, 30 seconds. Remove the pine nuts from the pan and set them aside.

2. Pour the olive oil into the saucepan. Add the onions and sauté until translucent, 3 minutes.

3. Add the quinoa and sauté with the onions for 2 minutes to toast.

4. Add the broth, bring the mixture to a boil, then cover and reduce the heat to low. Simmer for 10 to 12 minutes, until the liquid is almost fully absorbed.

5. Remove the pot from the heat and let it sit, covered, for 5 minutes to finish absorbing the liquid.

6. Stir in the pine nuts, tomatoes, parsley, and lemon juice. Serve immediately.

7. Store leftovers in the refrigerator for up to 2 to 3 days.

SIMPLE SWAP: Walnuts can be used in place of pine nuts. Toast the walnuts to enhance the nuttiness and texture of the dish.

PER SERVING: Calories: 279; Total fat: 15g; Saturated fat: 2g; Sodium: 46mg; Carbohydrates: 30g; Fiber: 4g; Protein: 7g; Calcium: 29mg; Potassium: 361mg

LOW-CALORIE MASHED POTATOES

5-INGREDIENT   EXTRA LOW CALORIE   ONE-POT
PREP TIME: 5 minutes   **COOK TIME:** 15 minutes
SERVES 6

Mashed potatoes always felt like so much work, until I learned it doesn't have to involve so many pieces of equipment. These mashed potatoes are all done in one pot, with no draining needed! The chicken broth and Greek yogurt provide flavor in place of traditional butter and cream, making these spuds a low-calorie comfort food.

2 pounds Yukon Gold potatoes, chopped into 1-inch cubes

1½ cups low-sodium chicken broth

¼ cup plain nonfat Greek yogurt

2 tablespoons chopped chives

Salt

Freshly ground black pepper

1. In a medium pot over high heat, add the chopped potatoes and chicken broth. Bring to a boil, uncovered. Once the liquid starts to boil, reduce the heat to medium-high, cover, and simmer for 10 minutes.

2. Remove the pot from the stove. Do not drain the liquid. Add the yogurt and chives and season with salt and pepper. Using a potato masher or fork, mash the potatoes to your desired texture.

3. Store leftover potatoes in a sealed container in the refrigerator for 3 to 5 days.

LOVE YOUR LEFTOVERS: Turn leftover mashed potatoes into potato pancakes by mixing 2 cups cold mashed potatoes with 2 large eggs and ¼ cup flour. Spoon ¼ cup batter onto a hot greased skillet and brown on both sides.

PER SERVING: Calories: 135; Total fat: 1g; Saturated fat: 0g; Sodium: 55mg; Carbohydrates: 28g; Fiber: 2g; Protein: 5g; Calcium: 33mg; Potassium: 698mg

ROSEMARY-PARMESAN SMASHED POTATOES

5-INGREDIENT   EXTRA LOW CALORIE

PREP TIME: 5 minutes   **COOK TIME:** 30 minutes

SERVES 4

Enjoy crispy smashed potatoes in a simple side dish that takes a plain baked potato to the next level. Softened potatoes are flattened then roasted with herb seasoning and Parmesan cheese for a crisp, savory texture. Change up your spuds by using a flavored olive oil, such as garlic-infused oil.

1 pound baby potatoes

2 tablespoons olive oil

1 teaspoon crushed dried rosemary

1 teaspoon salt

1 teaspoon freshly ground black pepper

1 tablespoon Parmesan cheese

1. Preheat the oven to 450°F. Line a sheet pan with parchment paper or nonstick aluminum foil.

2. Pierce the potatoes two or three times with a fork, then place them in a microwave-safe bowl and cook for 5 minutes on high until softened.

3. Line the potatoes on the sheet pan 2 to 3 inches apart. Using a potato masher or the bottom of a mug, gently press down on the potatoes to flatten. Drizzle the olive oil over them, then top with rosemary, salt, pepper, and Parmesan cheese. Roast for 20 to 25 minutes, until crispy.

4. Store leftover potatoes in the refrigerator for up to 4 days.

LOVE YOUR LEFTOVERS: Repurpose your leftovers by incorporating them into the Sheet Pan Veggie Hash (page 30).

PER SERVING: Calories: 152; Total fat: 7g; Saturated fat: 1g; Sodium: 611mg; Carbohydrates: 20g; Fiber: 3g; Protein: 3g; Calcium: 25mg; Potassium: 481mg

LEMON-SHALLOT CHAMPAGNE VINAIGRETTE

EXTRA LOW CALORIE   ONE-POT

PREP TIME: 10 minutes

MAKES 1 CUP

This simple dressing will add zing to any salad. It also can be drizzled over steamed or roasted vegetables for added flavor. Enjoy this dressing paired with Beet, Goat Cheese, and Pistachio Salad (page 43) and Grilled Halloumi Salad (page 46). Feel free to swap out the champagne vinegar for apple cider or white wine vinegar.

¼ cup champagne vinegar

1 tablespoon minced shallot

1 garlic clove, minced

1 teaspoon Dijon mustard

Zest and juice of ½ lemon

1 tablespoon fresh thyme, or
    1 teaspoon dried thyme

¾ cup extra-virgin olive oil

Salt

Freshly ground black pepper

1. In a small bowl, whisk together the vinegar, shallot, garlic, Dijon, lemon zest, lemon juice, and thyme.

2. Add the oil and season with salt and pepper. Whisk the ingredients together until combined.

3. Store the dressing in the refrigerator for up to 2 weeks.

COOKING HACK: Combine the dressing in a Mason jar and shake to blend, which cuts down on extra items to clean.

PER SERVING (2 TABLESPOONS): Calories: 183; Total fat: 20g; Saturated fat: 3g; Sodium: 47mg; Carbohydrates: 1g; Fiber: 0g; Protein: 0g; Calcium: 4mg; Potassium: 17mg

RASPBERRY–POPPY SEED DRESSING

5-INGREDIENT   EXTRA LOW CALORIE   ONE-POT
PREP TIME: 5 minutes
MAKES 1½ CUPS

Give your salads a sweet flavor and pop of color with a refreshing fruit-based dressing. This dressing is delicious in salads featuring fruits or roasted vegetables, enhancing their sweetness. Creating your own dressing cuts down on added sugars found in store-bought versions.

1 cup fresh or defrosted frozen raspberries

6 tablespoons red wine vinegar

2 tablespoons honey

1 teaspoon ground mustard powder

½ cup avocado oil

1 teaspoon poppy seeds

1. In a food processor or blender, combine the raspberries, vinegar, honey, and mustard powder. Pulse to blend until a liquid has formed.

2. Slowly drizzle the avocado oil into the mixture while processing to combine.

3. Pour the dressing into a sealed container. Add the poppy seeds and shake to combine.

4. Store the dressing in the refrigerator for up to 2 weeks.

SERVING SUGGESTION: Enjoy this dressing on the Roasted Delicata Squash, Cranberry, and Gorgonzola Salad (page 47) or dress a simple salad of spinach, strawberries, walnuts, and goat cheese.

PER SERVING (2 TABLESPOONS): Calories: 100; Total fat: 9g; Saturated fat: 1g; Sodium: 1mg; Carbohydrates: 4g; Fiber: 1g; Protein: 0g; Calcium: 7mg; Potassium: 23mg

AVOCADO BUTTERMILK RANCH DRESSING

EXTRA LOW CALORIE **ONE-POT**
PREP TIME: 5 minutes
MAKES 1½ CUPS

Cut back on the saturated fat and calories found in store-bought ranch dressings by creating your own low-calorie version with heart-healthy avocado and tangy buttermilk. This dressing goes great with salads and bowls such as the Sunflower Taco Salad Bowl (page 52) and Cauliflower Rice Burrito Bowl (page 49), and it even does double duty as a spread or dip.

1¼ cups low-fat buttermilk

1 medium ripe avocado, peeled, pitted, and halved

1 garlic clove

Juice of 1 lime

2 teaspoons onion powder

1 teaspoon dried chives

1 teaspoon dried parsley

1 teaspoon dried dill

½ teaspoon salt

½ teaspoon freshly ground black pepper

1. In a food processor or blender, combine the buttermilk, avocado, garlic, lime juice, onion powder, chives, parsley, dill, salt, and pepper. Pulse to blend until a smooth liquid has formed. Chill until ready to use.

2. Store the dressing in a sealed container in the refrigerator for up to 1 week.

SERVING SUGGESTION: Create crudités with fresh raw vegetables and this dressing as a dip for a tasty appetizer or snack.

PER SERVING (2 TABLESPOONS): Calories: 40; Total fat: 3g; Saturated fat: 0g; Sodium: 147mg; Carbohydrates: 3g; Fiber: 1g; Protein: 1g; Calcium: 37mg; Potassium: 132mg

SESAME, MISO, AND GINGER DRESSING

EXTRA LOW CALORIE   ONE-POT
PREP TIME: 5 minutes
MAKES 1 CUP

Top your salads or noodle bowls with this simple umami dressing. The miso paste adds gut-healthy probiotics, while the garlic and ginger deliver anti-inflammatory benefits. In addition to making a tasty salad dressing, this dressing can be tossed with steamed, roasted, or sautéed vegetables for a quick side dish.

2 tablespoons sesame oil

¼ cup avocado oil

3 tablespoons rice wine vinegar

2 tablespoons low-sodium soy sauce

1 garlic clove, quartered

1 (1-inch) piece fresh ginger, peeled and quartered (see Technique Trick)

1 tablespoon mirin or honey

1 tablespoon white miso

1 tablespoon sesame seeds

1. In a food processor or blender, combine the sesame oil, avocado oil, vinegar, soy sauce, garlic, ginger, mirin, and miso and puree until smooth. Transfer the dressing to a container and stir in the sesame seeds.

2. Store the dressing in the refrigerator for up to 3 to 4 weeks.

TECHNIQUE TRICK: Use a spoon to peel away the skin from fresh ginger.

PER SERVING (2 TABLESPOONS): Calories: 104; Total fat: 11g; Saturated fat: 1g; Sodium: 208mg; Carbohydrates: 1g; Fiber: 0g; Protein: 1g; Calcium: 4mg; Potassium: 24mg

SPINACH-PISTACHIO PESTO SAUCE

5-INGREDIENT   EXTRA LOW CALORIE   ONE-POT
PREP TIME: 10 minutes
MAKES ½ CUP

Most people are familiar with basil pesto, but there are many variations for this easy and delicious sauce. In this version, spinach increases the nutritional quality, and the pistachios provide a nutty flavor and texture along with protein. Pesto makes a great condiment, or try stirring some into recipes such as Savory Pesto Oats (page 27) and Low-Calorie Mashed Potatoes (page 134).

½ cup baby spinach, firmly packed

½ cup fresh basil, firmly packed

1 garlic clove

2 tablespoons water, plus more as needed

3 tablespoons grated Parmesan cheese

2 tablespoons shelled pistachios, toasted

3 tablespoons extra-virgin olive oil

1. In a food processor or blender, combine the spinach, basil, garlic, water, Parmesan cheese, and pistachios. Pulse to combine until a soft paste forms.

2. Slowly add in the oil while blending and pulse until your desired consistency is reached. If you prefer a thinner sauce, add an additional 1 to 2 tablespoons of water.

3. Store the sauce in the refrigerator for up to 5 days or freeze for up to 6 months.

SIMPLE SWAP: Any greens can work in this recipe, including kale, chard, arugula, and even the green tops of carrots. Most nuts or seeds can be used in place of the pistachios, including pine nuts, walnuts, cashews, sunflower seeds, and pepitas.

PER SERVING (1 TABLESPOON): Calories: 65; Total fat: 6g; Saturated fat: 1g; Sodium: 36mg; Carbohydrates: 1g; Fiber: 0g; Protein: 1g; Calcium: 23mg; Potassium: 40mg

TZATZIKI SAUCE

5-INGREDIENT   EXTRA LOW CALORIE   ONE-POT

PREP TIME: 5 minutes
MAKES 1¼ CUPS

This traditional Mediterranean sauce combines cucumbers, yogurt, herbs, and spices for a versatile dressing. Enjoy this sauce with a Falafel Bowl (page 51), drizzle as a topping for Lamb Tacos with Cucumber, Tomato, and Goat Cheese (page 121), or spread onto Spinach and Feta Lamb Burgers (page 122).

½ seedless English cucumber

1 cup plain nonfat
   Greek yogurt

1 tablespoon lemon juice

1 garlic clove

½ tablespoon extra-virgin
   olive oil

1 tablespoon fresh dill, or
   1 teaspoon dried dill

Salt

Freshly ground black pepper

1. Using a food processor or a box grater, grate the cucumber. Transfer the grated cucumber to a few pieces of layered paper towel, wrap the cucumber in it, and squeeze to remove any excess liquid. Transfer the cucumber to a small bowl.

2. In a food processor with a chopper attachment, combine the Greek yogurt, lemon juice, garlic, oil, and dill. Season with salt and pepper. Pulse to combine.

3. Add the dressing to the bowl with the cucumber and stir to combine. Chill until ready to use.

4. Store the sauce in a sealed container in the refrigerator for up to 3 days.

LOVE YOUR LEFTOVERS: Use leftover sauce as a dip with raw vegetables for a quick, healthy snack.

PER SERVING (2 TABLESPOONS): Calories: 24; Total fat: 1g; Saturated fat: 0g; Sodium: 24mg; Carbohydrates: 2g; Fiber: 0g; Protein: 3g; Calcium: 38mg; Potassium: 65mg

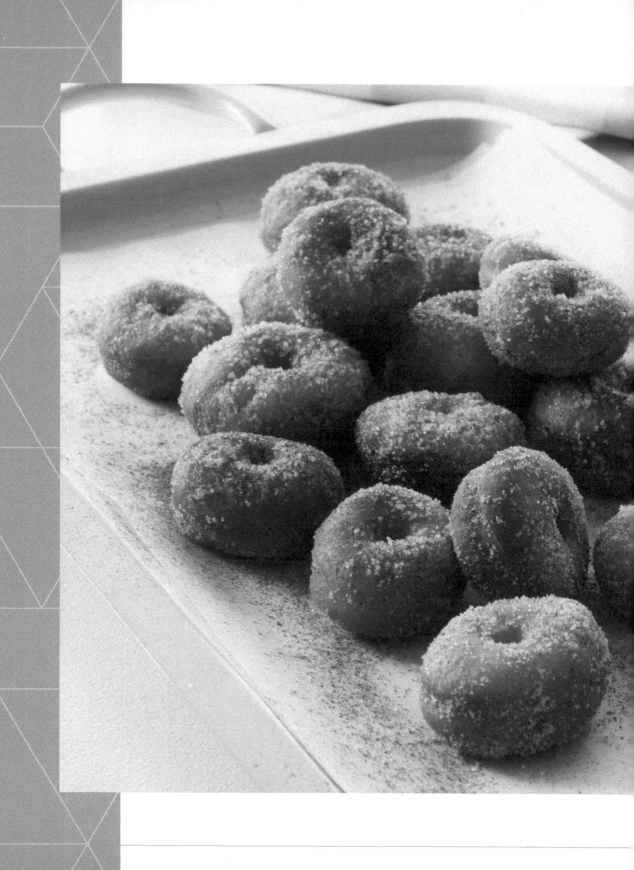

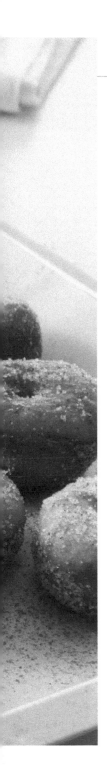

CHAPTER NINE

Yes, You Can Still Have Snacks and Dessert

Yes, you can in fact have snacks and desserts, and you don't even have to eat all your vegetables first. Let's distinguish between a "snack" and a "treat." Snacks are mini meals that get you through to your next main meal. They are nourishing for your body and keep energy and hunger levels in check. Treats are foods to enjoy on occasion, and denying yourself treats can ultimately lead to binge-fests and guilt. Instead, enjoy treats without guilt by having them on occasion and in moderation.

CRISPY BANANA SUSHI

5-INGREDIENT   EXTRA LOW CALORIE   ONE-POT

PREP TIME: 5 minutes
SERVES 1

Enjoy a simple but fancy snack by creating a "sushi roll" using a tortilla, banana, nut butter, and puffed rice cereal for extra crunch. You can even enjoy this banana sushi for a quick breakfast. Feel free to swap the almond butter for any nut or seed butter.

1 (6-inch) whole-wheat tortilla

1 tablespoon almond butter

2 tablespoons puffed
  rice cereal

1 banana, peeled and whole

Hemp seeds, for garnish
  (optional)

1. Lay a tortilla flat and spread the almond butter to coat the tortilla. Spread the puffed rice cereal over the almond butter, then place a whole banana at one end of the tortilla. Roll up the tortilla so the banana is tightly rolled inside with the almond butter and puffed rice cereal.

2. Cut the rolled tortilla into ¾-inch slices and arrange the sushi slices with the banana facing upward. Sprinkle hemp seeds on top and enjoy immediately.

SIMPLE SWAP: You can make this a chocolate treat by using chocolate-hazelnut spread or chocolate puffed rice cereal.

PER SERVING: Calories: 377; Total fat: 16g; Saturated fat: 3g; Sodium: 213mg, Carbohydrates: 56g; Fiber: 12g; Protein: 11g; Calcium: 170mg; Potassium: 869mg

PEA HUMMUS

5-INGREDIENT   EXTRA LOW CALORIE   ONE-POT
PREP TIME: 5 minutes
MAKES 1 CUP

Did you know hummus can be made with other legumes besides chickpeas? Peas are just one alternative. Peas provide a good source of fiber and protein in this snack dip or spread, plus they add a fun pop of color on your plate. Make a batch to enjoy as a quick snack during the workweek. Serve with raw vegetables, whole-grain crackers, or crostini.

1 cup frozen peas, thawed

2 tablespoons tahini

3 garlic cloves

2 tablespoons lemon juice

1 teaspoon red pepper flakes, plus more for garnish (optional)

¼ teaspoon kosher salt, plus more for garnish

¼ teaspoon freshly ground black pepper, plus more for garnish

2 tablespoons extra-virgin olive oil, plus more for garnish

1. In a food processor or blender, combine the peas, tahini, garlic, lemon juice, red pepper flakes (if using), salt, and pepper. Pulse to combine, occasionally scraping down the sides.

2. With the processor running, add the olive oil, 1 tablespoon at a time. Process until your desired consistency is reached.

3. When ready to serve, drizzle with additional olive oil, red pepper flakes (if using), salt, and pepper.

4. Store leftover hummus in the refrigerator for up to 1 week.

SIMPLE SWAP: Frozen or fresh shelled edamame can be used in place of the peas for another variation.

PER SERVING (2 TABLESPOONS): Calories: 69; Total fat: 5g; Saturated fat: 1g; Sodium: 78mg; Carbohydrates: 4g; Fiber: 1g; Protein: 2g; Calcium: 23mg; Potassium: 68mg

ALMOND-STUFFED DATES

5-INGREDIENT   EXTRA LOW CALORIE   ONE-POT

PREP TIME: 5 minutes

SERVES 4

Dates have a natural sweetness, plus they're loaded with protein, iron, and fiber. Enjoy a snack of pitted dates stuffed with almond butter and a fresh almond. Just purchase dates that are already pitted so you don't have to remove the pit yourself.

8 Medjool dates, dried and pitted

4 tablespoons almond butter

8 whole raw almonds

Sea salt, for garnish

Mini chocolate chips, for garnish

Ground cinnamon, for garnish

1. Create a lengthwise slit halfway through the dates. Spread ½ tablespoon of almond butter inside each date. Place an almond on top of the almond butter in the middle. Garnish with sea salt, chocolate chips, and ground cinnamon.

2. Store leftovers in a sealed container at room temperature for up to 1 week.

LOVE YOUR LEFTOVERS: Toss one or two stuffed dates into a smoothie, such as the Golden Milk Smoothie (page 24), for added sweetness and thickness.

PER SERVING: Calories: 245; Total fat: 10g; Saturated fat: 1g; Sodium: 40mg; Carbohydrates: 40g; Fiber: 5g; Protein: 5g; Calcium: 93mg; Potassium: 471mg

PARMESAN CRISPS

5-INGREDIENT   EXTRA LOW CALORIE   ONE-POT
PREP TIME: 10 minutes   **COOK TIME:** 5 minutes
SERVES 4

These Parmesan Crisps are my husband's favorite snack. With only a few ingredients, they're super simple to make. A great savory snack, these crisps are also delicious on top of salads, such as Kale Caesar Salad (page 41), or with soups, such as Tomato-Basil Soup (page 76) or Pumpkin and Pear Soup (page 77).

Nonstick cooking spray

1 (4-ounce) block Parmesan cheese

Freshly ground black pepper (optional)

1. Preheat the oven to 400°F. Line a sheet pan with parchment paper and spray it with cooking spray.

2. In a small bowl, finely grate the Parmesan cheese using the small holes on a box grater or a zester.

3. Use a tablespoon to create mounds of the Parmesan cheese on the parchment paper, then use the back side of the spoon to flatten out the mounds, keeping them at least 2 inches apart. Garnish with pepper (if using). Bake for 5 to 8 minutes, until golden.

4. Allow to cool before removing from the parchment paper. Enjoy immediately.

5. Store leftovers in a sealed container at room temperature for up to 3 days.

COOKING HACK: A fine grating attachment on a food processor can quickly grate the Parmesan cheese.

PER SERVING: Calories: 119; Total fat: 8g; Saturated fat: 4g; Sodium: 511mg; Carbohydrates: 4g; Fiber: 0g; Protein: 8g; Calcium: 242mg; Potassium: 51mg

AIR FRYER–ROASTED RANCH CHICKPEAS

EXTRA LOW CALORIE   ONE-POT
PREP TIME: 5 minutes   **COOK TIME:** 20 minutes
SERVES 2

Roasted chickpeas are a simple snack loaded with protein and fiber. They also make a crunchy swap for croutons on salads. The secret to crispy chickpeas is to dry them as much as possible before roasting. These chickpeas can also be cooked in a 400°F oven, but cooking time may take between 30 to 45 minutes.

1 (15.5-ounce) can chickpeas, drained and rinsed

2 tablespoons dry buttermilk powder (see Cooking Hack)

2 teaspoons dried parsley

2 teaspoons onion powder

1 teaspoon dried chives

½ teaspoon garlic powder

¼ teaspoon dried dill

¼ teaspoon salt

¼ teaspoon freshly ground black pepper

Nonstick cooking spray

1. Dry the chickpeas by spreading them out on a sheet pan lined with layers of paper towels. Pat dry with another layer of paper towels on top and then allow to air-dry for 5 minutes.

2. In a small bowl, make the ranch seasoning blend by combining the buttermilk powder, parsley, onion powder, chives, garlic powder, dill, salt, and pepper. Set aside.

3. Spray the basket of an air fryer with cooking spray. Spread the dry chickpeas in the basket and cook at 400°F for 5 minutes.

4. Toss the chickpeas, spray them with cooking spray, and cook for another 15 minutes, tossing every 5 minutes, until browned and crisp.

5. Toss the cooked chickpeas with 1 to 2 tablespoons of ranch seasoning blend and enjoy immediately.

6. Store leftover chickpeas in a sealed container at room temperature for up to 1 week. Store any leftover ranch seasoning in a sealed container to use with another batch of chickpeas.

COOKING HACK: Look for dry buttermilk powder in the baking aisle. You can also purchase a premade ranch seasoning blend or swap for a different seasoning, such as cinnamon sugar or salt and pepper.

PER SERVING: Calories: 201; Total fat: 4g; Saturated fat: 1g; Sodium: 569mg; Carbohydrates: 32g; Fiber: 8g; Protein: 11g; Calcium: 142mg; Potassium: 272mg

S'MORES YOGURT PARFAIT

5-INGREDIENT   EXTRA LOW CALORIE   ONE-POT

PREP TIME: 5 minutes

SERVES 2

Who doesn't love a s'more? That combo of chocolate, graham cracker, and marshmallows is such a comfort food. Boost up the nutrition of your traditional s'more by turning it into a parfait with Greek yogurt. Vanilla or chocolate yogurt can be used as the base, layered with crushed graham crackers, chocolate chips, and mini marshmallows.

2 graham cracker
  sheets, crushed

1 cup vanilla or chocolate
  Greek yogurt

¼ cup chocolate chips

½ cup mini marshmallows

1. In two 8-ounce glasses or Mason jars, layer the crushed graham crackers, yogurt, chocolate chips, and marshmallows. Repeat 1 or 2 more times.

2. Store leftover parfaits in the refrigerator for up to 2 days.

TECHNIQUE TRICK: Want to give your marshmallows a toast? Use a culinary butane torch to brown the top layer of marshmallows.

PER SERVING: Calories: 311; Total fat: 11g; Saturated fat: 6g; Sodium: 141mg; Carbohydrates: 48g; Fiber: 2g; Protein: 9g; Calcium: 206mg; Potassium: 371mg

PINEAPPLE-BANANA WHIP

5-INGREDIENT   EXTRA LOW CALORIE   ONE-POT

PREP TIME: 5 minutes

SERVES 2

This frozen pineapple-banana "nice cream" will remind you of vacation or summertime. A high-powered food processor or blender is key to whipping the frozen fruit into a smooth, creamy texture. I don't anticipate you will have leftovers, but if you do, you can store leftover whip in ice cube trays in the freezer and add it to smoothies.

1 cup frozen pineapple chunks

1 frozen banana

2½ teaspoons confectioners' sugar

½ cup unsweetened canned coconut milk

In a food processor or high-powered blender, combine the pineapple, banana, sugar, and coconut milk. Blend, scraping down the sides or using the tamper of a blender to push down the ingredients to combine, until it achieves a creamy consistency. Enjoy immediately.

COOKING HACK: For a thicker consistency, store the coconut milk can upside down in your pantry, then use the milk solids only.

PER SERVING: Calories: 217; Total fat: 12g; Saturated fat: 11g; Sodium: 9mg; Carbohydrates: 29g; Fiber: 3g; Protein: 2g; Calcium: 24mg; Potassium: 426mg

AIR-FRYER CINNAMON-SUGAR DONUTS

5-INGREDIENT EXTRA LOW CALORIE ONE-POT
PREP TIME: 10 minutes **COOK TIME:** 10 minutes
SERVES 8

Several donut shops have popped up near my home recently, completely changing everything I previously knew about donuts. What I do know about donuts is that they are treats, and handmade donuts should be savored. I've also learned that you can create your own donuts using an air fryer. Alternatively, bake them at 375°F for 10 to 15 minutes—using a sheet pan with a rack will help the air circulate and crisp the donuts.

1 (16-ounce) can refrigerated jumbo flaky biscuits

½ cup sugar

½ tablespoon ground cinnamon

Nonstick cooking spray

4 tablespoons (½ stick) unsalted butter, melted

1. Separate the biscuits. Using a 1-inch round biscuit cutter, cut out the center of each biscuit.

2. In a shallow bowl, combine the sugar and cinnamon and set aside.

3. Spray the basket of an air fryer with cooking spray, then place the biscuit donuts in the air fryer basket in a single layer. Cook at 350°F for 5 minutes, until browned, flipping halfway through.

4. Repeat with the remaining dough. You can also cook the donut holes for a total of 3 minutes, turning halfway through.

5. Remove the donuts from the air fryer and place on a plate. Brush the melted butter on the cooked donuts, then roll the donuts in the cinnamon-sugar mixture. Enjoy immediately.

6. Cover leftover donuts with plastic wrap for 1 to 2 days at room temperature or up to 5 days in the refrigerator. Reheat in the air fryer or a toaster oven at 350°F for 2 to 3 minutes.

TECHNIQUE TRICK: If you don't have a biscuit cutter, use the mouth of a bottle or an apple corer, or simply use a paring knife to cut out a hole in the middle.

PER SERVING: Calories: 254; Total fat: 10g; Saturated fat: 6g; Sodium: 498mg; Carbohydrates: 38g; Fiber: 2g; Protein: 4g; Calcium: 22mg; Potassium: 94mg

APPLE CRISP

5-INGREDIENT   EXTRA LOW CALORIE

PREP TIME: 10 minutes   **COOK TIME:** 20 minutes

SERVES 4

I love making a homemade apple pie, but it's a ton of work. There are only two people in my home, so a whole pie is a lot. I created these Apple Crisps instead, making individual portions using ramekins. They come together quick for a warm after-dinner treat or holiday dessert. Serve topped with Greek yogurt or a scoop of vanilla ice cream for à la mode goodness.

2 apples, peeled, cored, and thinly sliced

¾ cup rolled oats

3 tablespoons unsalted butter, cold

2 tablespoons maple syrup

½ teaspoon ground cinnamon

1. Preheat the oven to 400°F. Lightly grease a pie pan or four ramekins and place the apple slices in the pan or ramekins.

2. Place the oats in a medium bowl. Cut the butter into the oats using a pastry blender until the butter is the size of peas. Stir in the maple syrup and cinnamon. Spread the topping over the apples and bake for 20 minutes, until the topping is browned. Serve warm.

3. Store leftover crisp tightly wrapped in the refrigerator for up to 1 week. Reheat in a 350°F oven for 10 to 15 minutes, until heated through.

TECHNIQUE TRICK: If you don't have a pastry blender, you can cut the butter into small pieces and use a fork to mash the butter with the oats. You can also combine the oats and small pieces of cold butter in a food processor and pulse a few times until it achieves a crumbly texture.

PER SERVING: Calories: 242; Total fat: 10g; Saturated fat: 6g; Sodium: 4mg; Carbohydrates: 35g; Fiber: 5g; Protein: 4g; Calcium: 34mg; Potassium: 223mg

CHICKPEA-TAHINI BLONDIES

EXTRA LOW CALORIE

PREP TIME: 5 minutes   **COOK TIME:** 25 minutes

SERVES 6

I may be a brownie fan at heart, but as a blonde girl, I'm always out to prove that blondes can have more fun—even in baked good form! These fudgy blondies are loaded with fiber and protein—not something often associated with treats. Even my husband had to be convinced these are made with chickpeas because he couldn't tell the difference.

Nonstick cooking spray

⅓ cup rolled oats

1 (15.5-ounce) can chickpeas, drained and rinsed

½ cup tahini

⅓ cup maple syrup

2 teaspoons vanilla extract

¼ teaspoon salt

¼ teaspoon baking powder

¼ teaspoon baking soda

½ cup chocolate chips

1. Preheat the oven to 350ºF. Grease an 8-by-8-inch baking dish with cooking spray.

2. In a food processor or blender, pulse the oats until they form a flour. Remove the oat flour from the food processor and set aside.

3. In the same food processor, add the chickpeas, tahini, maple syrup, and vanilla and blend until combined.

4. Add the oat flour, salt, baking powder, and baking soda and blend again to combine, scraping down the sides.

5. Stir in the chocolate chips by hand, then transfer the batter to the prepared baking dish. Bake for 20 to 25 minutes, until the edges are browned and a toothpick inserted into the center comes out clean. Cool completely before slicing into pieces to enjoy.

6. Store leftovers in a sealed container at room temperature for up to 5 days or freeze for up to 3 months.

SIMPLE SWAP: Any nut or seed butter can be swapped for the tahini.

PER SERVING: Calories: 311; Total fat: 17g; Saturated fat: 5g; Sodium: 259mg; Carbohydrates: 35g; Fiber: 6g; Protein: 8g; Calcium: 140mg; Potassium: 290mg

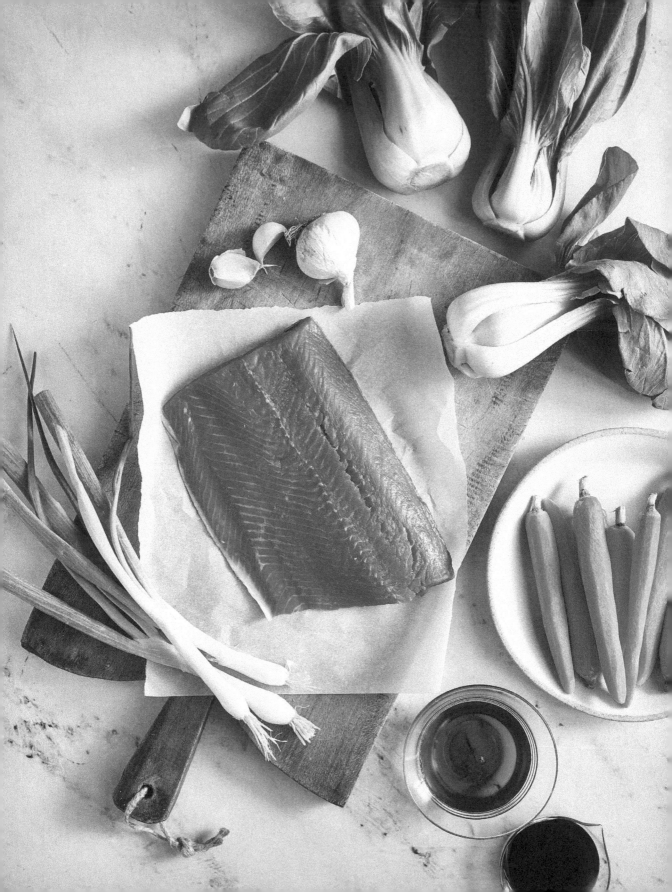

MEASUREMENT CONVERSIONS

VOLUME EQUIVALENTS	U.S. STANDARD	U.S. STANDARD (OUNCES)	METRIC (APPROXIMATE)
LIQUID	2 tablespoons	1 fl. oz.	30 mL
	¼ cup	2 fl. oz.	60 mL
	½ cup	4 fl. oz.	120 mL
	1 cup	8 fl. oz.	240 mL
	1½ cups	12 fl. oz.	355 mL
	2 cups or 1 pint	16 fl. oz.	475 mL
	4 cups or 1 quart	32 fl. oz.	1 L
	1 gallon	128 fl. oz.	4 L
DRY	⅛ teaspoon	—	0.5 mL
	¼ teaspoon	—	1 mL
	½ teaspoon	—	2 mL
	¾ teaspoon	—	4 mL
	1 teaspoon	—	5 mL
	1 tablespoon	—	15 mL
	¼ cup	—	59 mL
	⅓ cup	—	79 mL
	½ cup	—	118 mL
	⅔ cup	—	156 mL
	¾ cup	—	177 mL
	1 cup	—	235 mL
	2 cups or 1 pint	—	475 mL
	3 cups	—	700 mL
	4 cups or 1 quart	—	1 L
	½ gallon	—	2 L
	1 gallon	—	4 L

OVEN TEMPERATURES

FAHRENHEIT	CELSIUS (APPROXIMATE)
250°F	120°C
300°F	150°C
325°F	165°C
350°F	180°C
375°F	190°C
400°F	200°C
425°F	220°C
450°F	230°C

WEIGHT EQUIVALENTS

U.S. STANDARD	METRIC (APPROXIMATE)
½ ounce	15 g
1 ounce	30 g
2 ounces	60 g
4 ounces	115 g
8 ounces	225 g
12 ounces	340 g
16 ounces or 1 pound	455 g

RESOURCES

Mandy Enright, The FOOD + MOVEMENT® Dietitian (MandyEnright.com): My website containing information on nutrition, recipes, fitness, and mindfulness.

MyPlate (MyPlate.gov): Learn how to assemble healthy meals that focus on variety, balance, and moderation.

National Dairy Council (USDairy.com): A nonprofit organization that provides science-based education on the benefits of dairy foods.

Oldways (OldwaysPT.org): A nonprofit organization helping people rediscover, learn, and enjoy the healthy, sustainable joys of the "old ways" of eating.

Produce for Better Health (FruitsandVeggies.org): A nonprofit organization committed to encouraging people to eat more fruits and vegetables every day.

Seafood Nutrition Partnership (SeafoodNutrition.org): A nonprofit organization working to inspire a healthier America and raise awareness about the nutritional benefits of eating seafood.

Tomato Wellness (TomatoWellness.com): An organization dedicated to supporting research, awareness, and education about canned tomato products.

US Food and Drug Administration (FDA.gov/food/new-nutrition-facts-label /how-understand-and-use-nutrition-facts-label): Further information on reading and interpreting food labels.

REFERENCES

American Psychological Association. "Why Do Dieters Regain Weight? Calorie Deprivation Alters Body and Mind, Overwhelming Willpower." Accessed December 19, 2020. APA.org/science/about/psa/2018/05/calorie-deprivation.

Hall, Kevin D., and Scott Kahan. "Maintenance of Lost Weight and Long-Term Management of Obesity." *Medical Clinics of North America* 102, no. 1 (January 2018): 183–197. DOI.org/10.1016/j.mcna.2017.08.012.

INDEX

ACKNOWLEDGMENTS

This book would not have been possible without the unending support from my husband, Joe. Thank you for the late-night brainstorming sessions, endless recipe testing, and last-minute trips to the grocery store because "I forgot this one thing."

To my friends, near and far, who helped test and taste-test recipes, you truly have my heart.

And finally, to my mom, who is responsible for getting me in the kitchen early in life. I still remember standing on a chair while helping because I was too short to reach the countertop. You and Dad have always supported me 100 percent.

Thank you to the team at Callisto Media for helping me with my first book-writing experience—I would've been lost without your guidance!

ABOUT THE AUTHOR

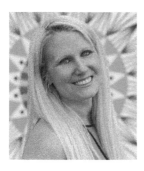

Mandy Enright, MS, RDN, RYT, is a registered dietitian, yoga and fitness instructor, speaker, and spokesperson. She specializes in corporate wellness, nutrition communications, and helping provide simple, actionable mealtime solutions from planning to preparation. A prior career as an advertising executive fuels her mission for promoting self-care to busy professionals. Mandy is known as the FOOD + MOVEMENT® Dietitian for her fun and flexible approach to maximize body and mind performance through lifestyle and mindset changes that integrate rather than deviate from our busy daily lives. She has been featured in national media outlets including *Today's Dietitian*, *U.S. News & World Report*, *Bridal Guide*, Livestrong, *Reader's Digest*, and the Food Network.

When not changing the health of corporate America, Mandy can be found exploring her home at the Jersey Shore with her husband, Joe, and their cavalier, Shiva the Diva. Learn more about Mandy at MandyEnright.com and follow her @MandyEnrightRD on Facebook, Twitter, Instagram, Pinterest, YouTube, and TikTok.

CPSIA information can be obtained
at www.ICGtesting.com
Printed in the USA
JSHW051219040521
14184JS00002B/3

9 781648 766558